'Wonderfully Strange'

by

Becky Shaw

'Wonderfully Strange'

by

Becky Shaw

Copyright © 2009

All rights reserved. No part of this publication may be reproduced, stored in a retrieval system or transmitted in any form or by any means electronic, mechanical, audio, visual or otherwise, without prior permission of the copyright owner. Nor can it be circulated in any form of binding or cover other than that in which it is published and without similar conditions including this condition being imposed on the subsequent purchaser.

ISBN: 978-0-9559591-0-3

Published by Becky Shaw in conjunction with Writersworld Ltd

Printed and bound by www.printondemand-worldwide.com

www.writersworld.co.uk

WRITERSWORLD
2 Bear Close
Woodstock
Oxfordshire
OX20 1JX
United Kingdom

- If you've ever been 'labelled'

- If you've ever worried about using mental health services

- If you've ever wondered how you'd cope if someone you know has mental health problems—then this book is for you.

Becky Shaw has successfully survived her own long journey through the mental health system.

As someone labelled psychotic, bulimic and a depressive she knows at first hand how it feels to be adrift in a system which she didn't understand and which didn't address her needs.

After years of feeling an outsider, Becky is now an established author with contributions to academic journals and books.

Her experience has given her a passion to help others who've had problems in dealing with mental health issues.

This book is an account of her journey through the system, plus practical help on how to manage, where to go and how to survive.

Introduction

I have used personally, and worked voluntarily, in the mental health services for 16 years. My background is in research and education. I teach within a variety of settings including the School of Nursing at Nottingham University and the Clinical Psychology department at Nottingham Trent and Leicester Universities. For 15 years I have run a mental health self-help group which helps support others experiencing mental health distress, on their road to recovery. I was one of the original reviewers for the Health Care Commission and I have carried out reviews for the joint reviews for CSCI (Commission for Social Care Inspection). I have led research and evaluation projects, including those for mental health media and independent research in education, within a variety of organisations. My current projects include leading a research team as chief investigator looking into the experience of using the Crisis Resolution and Home Treatment teams within Nottinghamshire and Leicestershire mental health trusts.

It was a nurse at a unit who described me as 'Wonderfully Strange.'

I don't know if it was intended as a compliment but I do know it's a description of me that fits. It sums me up well. I have a different outlook on life: but I am wonderful and I am loved.

It's taken me a long time to accept that I am a worthwhile and loveable human being, so for a long time I didn't accept the wonderful part either.

We all have parts of us that are different. The very fact that we're human makes each of us unique and wonderful.

I found from being a young child that I was different. I remember one phrase someone said to me when I was about five; "It's okay to be different!"

Maybe taking that literally was my downfall. I've had to learn to make choices and conform in some ways. But I do believe that being 'different' shouldn't stop me achieving because of my difference.

We live in a social world. Where there is difference between us there is room for conflict. What I want to propose is that acceptance in this world means accepting the differences in ourselves and others.

Thank you for taking the time to read this book. I hope it gives you a glimpse into my world and my experience. The more we share our experiences, the easier it will become to increase acceptance of difference.

Bit by bit people like me are writing, performing, teaching, singing and shouting out loud that things need to change.

We are human. *And we are you.*

One in four people suffers from some form of mental health problem at some point in their life. Despite better medication, better housing, and all the other conveniences of modern life there will always be families in crisis. There will always be those individuals who are more vulnerable than others. There will always be a need for a system that cares for those with mental health problems.

This book is to help produce a system that works. I wanted to write this book for myself and for you. Whether you're in the mental health system, supporting someone in the system, or working in the system, I hope this book will help you understand.

Anyone who has been 'labelled' needs to be treated as a human being. They may seem different but they still deserve respect, dignity and to be treated as someone able to make a contribution. You can still see them as having potential and strength, not simply as 'a problem' to be fixed, passed on or even worse, shelved.

I'm not here to dwell on the past. What's done is done. I include entries from diaries I've written in the past only to help you understand. They aren't great literature. Some of them were written when I was in severe distress. But I hope they will help show you what those of us with mental health problems go through on a daily basis.

What I want to focus on now is making positive change for the future. As a human being I know I'll continue to make mistakes, but that's okay. Some of our greatest lessons are learned from our mistakes.

In the first section of the book I look at some of the labels and show you what happened to me. In the second section of the book I'm offering a guide to the Mental Health Services in down-to-earth terms.

In Section 3 I look at help from outside the system.

Understanding the system is confusing for those in it, those supporting them and, dare I say it, even for those working in it. I'm not saying that if you have mental health issues you might not need help for the rest of your life. It depends on your problem. I accept I will need help for the long term. However, being in crisis and use of the mental health system can be shortened and less traumatic with the right information and support.

How you start off in the system often dictates what happens to you. If you know you have choices then it might make your life easier and your journey time shorter to find the help you need.

Wherever you are at the moment I hope that *you* can gain something from this book.

"If I can help someone else to believe that, despite their mental health issues they are a valid and valued human being, then writing this book will have the result I want."

Becky Shaw

Editor's comments

My first surprise on meeting Becky was when I commented on a plaster on her arm and she replied that she self-harmed. Maybe my reaction or lack of it was one of the factors that led to her contacting me several months later to ask if I would help her write her own book.

Becky and I discussed what she wanted her book to be about and who it was aimed at. She'd already written quite a lot about her experiences in the form of a diary and other pieces, so we met and together worked out a structure for the book, based on what she hoped it would achieve.

Then I began in the way I always do, by looking at what she already had and how it would fit into the structure. At that stage it was probably no more to me than a typical project. It quickly became quite other than a typical project as I was drawn into Becky's experiences and worked on how best to represent these to a reader who has no understanding of the mental health system.

Becky is a remarkable person. Whatever you think of her experiences, they have happened and she writes about them with honesty in this book. Working with her has taught me about people who I might in the past have thought of as 'different'. What I understand better than before is that they aren't 'others', they are you and me.

Becky states that she believes anyone given the right circumstances can suffer from mental health problems. I think she's right. However strong-minded or stable we are, in circumstances of deprivation, hunger, isolation or discrimination, we can become vulnerable. The people we think of as 'others' may have had life experiences which we also could find difficult to deal with.

Becky and I have both made journeys writing this book, individual and shared. We discussed the system, the therapies, the language, the help and lack of it and in exploring many of these topics have both grown. I've tried to pay Becky the compliment of treating her as I would any client—expecting things of her, setting deadlines and going for the best end-product we can get.

For my part it's been a privilege to work with Becky and I hope that what we've produced will help you understand in a way you didn't before.

Eileen Parr 2008

Acknowledgements

A book doesn't happen all by itself, so this is an appropriate place to acknowledge the people who've helped me to turn my dream into a reality.

To my Mum and Dad and all my family who have been there through thick and thin, who have supported me in every way, and for whom the word thank you will never be enough. Writing this book has been hard for me and hard for all my family but I hope through this book the mental health system can change, so thank you both for your contribution and for your support in this process. Being a parent is never easy and even harder when your own daughter is unwell, but you have both done the best anyone could and I hope that one day when I have children I can also support them like you have supported me.

To James; you see me for who I am, you believe in who I can be and you support me in ways that enable me to be at my best. Thank you for just being you.

To my editor, Eileen, who has encouraged me throughout the whole process, helped me believed it was possible and kept me steady when I wobbled. If you have a book you want to make happen but need support with, I can't think of anyone better to help you. See her website www.words-for-you.co.uk for more information.

To my illustrator, Brick, thank you for your support and advice in producing my book. Your drawings for my book really bring it to life. Brick has a website which I encourage you all to have a look at. www.brickbats.co.uk

To Graham, Sue and Charles at Writersworld, thank you all for helping me produce my book and for your patience and support.

During the last few months before publication I was extremely unwell. Your understanding during this difficult time was much appreciated. It has been lovely working with you all and I would recommend you to anyone thinking of writing their own book.

To Dawn, a nurse, and the first person to treat me as an equal and valuable human being, thank you.

To my friends, who have stood by me, including Keith, Claire, Polly and Paula.

To the workers who have supported me and my decisions, especially Nick J, Paul P, Karen H, Lyn and Jayne S.

To all those I work and have worked with, especially my research group and co-trainers.

To all my fellow peers at my support group who, although they would argue with this sentiment, have helped me far more than I have helped them.

I started to write a list of everyone I wanted to thank for being supportive throughout my life, but I quickly realised there were far too many people to thank individually. It was lovely to realise that people cared, and I am sad that I cannot possibly acknowledge everyone. So this is for all of you who have supported me, believed in me, been there for me just by being yourselves, and cared about me with all my strange quirks and difficulties.

Finally, to both my Grans, as although you are not here with me in the flesh, you will always be with me deep inside, and I could not finish this book without acknowledging you both and the contributions you have made. Both of you believed in me, laughed with me and cried with me and I will be forever grateful for all you have given me.

Dedication to my Grans

To my Grans
So wanted
A love
So true
You might need me
But I also need you
For a humour
And a love
That works both ways
We will be near
Till the end
Of our days

Becky

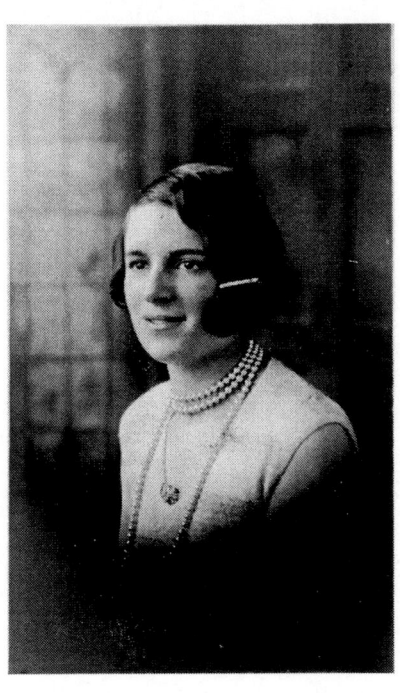

**Elsie Gould
(nee Bee)**

Born 27th December 1910
Died 3rd January 2008
97 years

(Seamstress/Upholstery machinist)

Full of fun and laughter and always had a smile for everyone

**Hilda Jean Shaw
(nee Plaistow)**

Born 25th February 1914
Died 25th June 2006
92 years

(Secretary/Shorthand typist)

Telegraph Crossword whiz kid

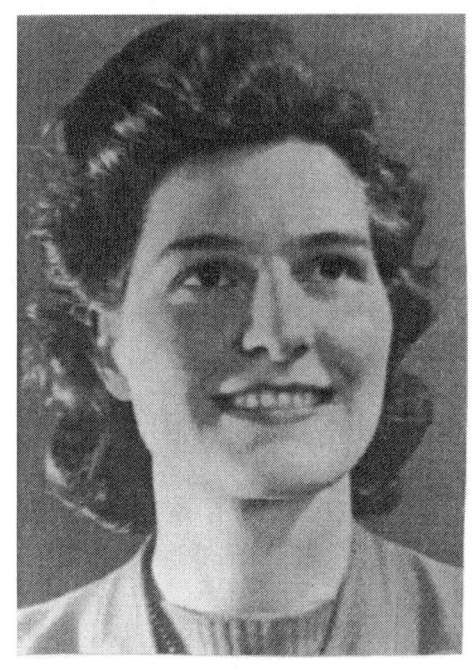

Contents

Introduction

Editor's comments

Section 1: My Journey   1
- Labelling   7
- Abnormality   15
- Abuse   23
- Exclusion & Isolation   29
- Agoraphobia   35
- Depression   37
- Bulimia   43
- Self-harm   47
- Suicide   53
- Psychosis   59

Section 2: The Mental Health System   75
- Statistics and Standards   77
- Available therapies in the Mental Health system   80
- The Mental Health Continuum   83
- Maslow and the hierarchy of needs   85
- My first encounter with the Mental Health system   91
- Diagnosis and medication   93
- The acute ward   97
- Current crisis provision   107

Workers in the Mental Health Service	114
Mental Health Service education	117

Section 3: Support outside the system — 125

Family	125
Friends	130
Support groups	132
Parents' perspective	135

Section 4: Recovery — 143

Relapse and crisis	146
Visit to Nigeria and its repercussions	149
My future	154
Final tips	159
Visions	160

Section 5: Glossary — 161

Section 6: Resources — 165

Rebecca Shaw Publications	171

References — 172

Why I need to publish this book — 174

Disclaimer

This book is one person's experience and view of the system.

Any information contained in it does not set out to replace medical and therapeutic treatment.

If you feel that you or someone close to you is suffering from depression or any other form of mental distress—ask for help. The sooner you receive the help you need the sooner you will start the process of recovery.

If you do not know where to begin to get help and don't want to involve your GP or family, then one of the national self-help groups such as Mind can offer you someone to talk to. See Section 6 for more information.

Section One

My journey

Where my journey started

A child's eye view of being different

I was brought up in a loving family and it may sound odd, but that led to some of the problems I faced. They wrapped me in cotton wool and protected me to such an extent that even by the time I went to university I hadn't caught a bus on my own or cooked for myself.

When I was a child I spent a lot of time with my grandmother who helped at the local village playgroup. I found it easier being around adults than other children. In school I was friendlier with the teachers than with the other children.

My only friend at school was somebody who abused my caring nature, my need to please her and my distress when I had not. I now know she did it for fun and that, because I was so upset at her shouting at me, she did it more.

My friends were the elderly of the village, not the young. I was bullied and tormented by the other school children. I was different. I cared about others, about trying my best and I understood right from wrong. I grew quickly and was adult before my time. I remember a lot about my past and childhood—little things about how I first discovered how to get out of my cot, the hours spent with the cantankerous cat, Soapie, time spent on my own, painting, and my Mum's frustration that I had few friends.

I remember my shiny black patent shoes that as soon as I had a single scratch I wanted a new pair. In fact I never had as many new pairs as I thought as my Dad just cleaned them up and put them back in the box.

Oh, and there's my goldfish, Flatter, who lived until I was 14 years old—but didn't. I won him at the Goose Fair and put him in a bowl at home that made him look flat, hence the name Flatter. When he developed a fan tail I thought he had matured, and I thought that he shed his skin like a snake and that is why he changed every few years. I was distraught when I found that he didn't—it was Flatter the 10th that was in the bowl! When he died I buried him in a plastic carton of water with some food, and was never fooled again.

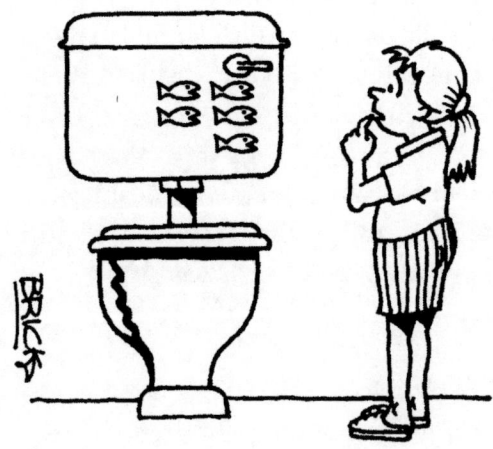

The causes of the distress I suffer lie in the roots of my past, through emotional and physical abuse. I now, however, have a future, and although I have my difficulties I give back what I can through voluntary work and in helping my peer support group. This also gives my life meaning and purpose, something a lot of us take for granted as I certainly did before I became acutely unwell. This also gives me a reason to live and a love of life again, especially when I am on an 'up' day.

How does mental health distress affect me?

Recurrent clinical depression, psychosis, self-harm, bulimia and anxiety are the main symptoms of the mental health distress I experience.

Life varies from day to day and week to week. Some days I feel I can conquer the world and other days I can barely bring myself to make a cup of tea or find the energy to get out of bed. I manage my life on how I am feeling and I am getting better at telling when I should stop and take a break. Sometimes this might mean stopping altogether and going for respite. At other times it might mean a few days or hours resting and taking time for me. If I did not manage my up-and-down life in this way I would become acutely unwell and end up back on a mental health acute ward, or worse—dead.

The cost of mental health problems in our society

The 'World Health Report 1999' demonstrates that neuropsychiatric conditions are the commonest cause of premature death and years of life loss. Besides the immense cost in personal and family suffering, mental illness costs in the region of £32 billion in England each year. This includes almost £12 billion in lost employment and approaching £8 billion in benefits payments.
(National Mental Health Service Framework, p14).

Mental health statistics

- One person in four people in the world will suffer from a mental health problem at some point in their life. (WHO 2001).

- Mental health problems account for up to a third of all GP consultations in Europe (WHO 2003).

- Estimates vary, but research suggests that 20% of children will have a mild mental health problem in any given year (Lifetime Impacts: Childhood and Adolescent Mental Health).

- Between 8% and 12% of the population experience anxiety or depression in any year (The Office for National Statistics Psychiatric Morbidity report, 2001). Fewer than 60% of them are employed on a full or part-time basis.

- Of the working population, only 17% of people with a diagnosis of serious mental illness are economically active.

- 1 in 5 people with mental health problems, particularly those with schizophrenia or bipolar disorder, make a major contribution to society by working in a voluntary capacity.

- In 2004, more than 5,500 people in the UK died by suicide. (Samaritans' suicide statistics).

- The UK has one of the highest rates of self-harm in Europe, at 400 per 100,000 population (Self-poisoning and self-injury in adults, Clinical Medicine, 2002).

- Suicide is in the top 10 causes of death in every country (WHO 2000).

Co-morbidity and mental health

Co-morbidity is the tendency of some groups of people to die earlier than the general population. People with mental health problems have a death rate that is 2.4 times higher then the general population.

The Bazelon Center for Mental Health Law (2004) found the following facts that were found to be prevalent in people who have a serious and persistent mental illness:

- Between 40% and 56% have a physical problem
- 35% have at least one undiagnosed medical disorder
- They are twice as likely to have multiple medical disorders (26% -vs- 12%)
- 42% have a physical health problem severe enough to limit their daily functioning
- Their HIV infection rates are 8 times as prevalent as in the general U.S. population
- 40% have co-occurring substance abuse disorders or substance dependence diagnoses
- 93% have visual problems
- 78% have auditory problems
- 60% have dental problems
- Their Hepatitis B rates are 5 times as prevalent and their Hepatitis C rates are 11 times the national average
- People with mental illness make up 44% of the U.S. tobacco market
- Obesity rates for adults with a mental illness are significantly higher (23.4%) than for adults without a mental illness (14.9%)

Labelling

Stigma and discrimination are parts of my life. I face them every day. You may not understand, and I don't expect you to empathise with my difficulties, such as the problem I often have even getting out of the house each day, but reading my story may help you to accept and support others you know who may have similar problems.

I could be your sister, or cousin, or friend.

One in four people trying to deal with their mental health problems means there are a lot of people out there in distress. Yet it's still seen as something not to be talked about, as something bad that you might catch, so *don't go near them*.

My friends describe me as lovable and fun. I don't carry an axe around with me. I've never been a risk in my life to anyone but myself. You're more likely to be at risk from the drunken youth in the city centre on a Friday night.

In this high-achieving, focused society, it's seen as a sign of weakness even to admit to stress. The thought of admitting to more severe mental health problems shuts many sufferers off from the people who can help them.

There is an ongoing debate about reducing the benefit budget and making sure only the 'deserving' receive money. I can only speak for myself, but with my health problems I know that benefits are vital for me.

Diary: December 2003

"Being on benefits is security, both financially and emotionally. However, being on benefits is also a trap, and demoralizing. I feel like a second-rate citizen because I am not earning and working like others; instead I am taking. I feel like the scum of the earth.

But I do have a part-time paid job for a few weeks of the year. It is paid very well and I have to come off benefits when I do it. It feels really good not to be reliant for that week on state handouts, although it's hard work and makes me ill afterwards.

Although I've never had a full-time paid job I believe I have made a valuable contribution to the community. I have worked in schools as a student. I have done lots of voluntary jobs and am still a volunteer. I set up and continue to run a support group for people with mental health difficulties.

I also help carry out audits, research and training in mental health."

Diary: June 2004

*"Having a label is more than a set of words written on a piece of paper; it's a label for life and it affects everything. Now that I have become ill my world has crumbled beneath me. Everything I had wanted to do in life — the teaching career, degree, a job, **a life** — has gone in one fell swoop!"*

It was only a matter of weeks before I had to be admitted to the psychiatric acute ward for the first time. That admission led to the longest and hardest six months of my life.

The mental health system takes everything away from you and things you at first could easily manage, become impossible.

I believe the mental health system is now synonymous with *institutionalisation* within the community—the asylums may be gone but the culture is still there. Workers don't believe you are capable human beings in many respects or do not realise that once upon a time, before you were ill, you had a life.

Diary: June 2004

"Saw my psychologist. I knew what I wanted to talk to him about today— my diagnosis of borderline personality disorder which I disagree with. He said that they have to put a label on me and he thought that it would 'suddenly disappear' off my records in few years with no reason given."

Half an hour to give me a label and five years to take it off!

He went on to say that a lot of symptoms suggestive of mental health problems could be applied to someone reacting in a completely normal way. There have been many studies that have shown this, where people have been admitted to a ward, behaved as normal and then been labelled *abnormal*.

It may seem odd to compare myself to a celebrity or pop star, but the same thing often happens to them. If they get into trouble, that incident goes on their press file, and even if they later have no trouble whatsoever, it will continue to come up in interviews as something that happened. It's a lazy, shorthand way for people to deal with someone/something they don't know about.

In exactly the same way, a label for a person with mental health problems is shorthand for workers in the system, their family and maybe the police if they come into contact.

Becoming an adult and spending years locked into the mental health system reinforced my ideas that I was somehow different, wrong and needed locking up so that I was hidden from society. Is this because other people can't cope with me or am I so deranged that I can't live a life with ordinary people?

Or is it not me but other people who have a fear that we all carry big axes to chop off their heads? I for one have never met a single mental health patient who owns an axe, never mind used one. I have, however, met a lot of people experiencing distress, fearful that their 'label' will be known to the outside world with the repercussions on their life that would follow.

I don't blame people for being scared of the unknown. It takes time to find out that we don't go around killing people, that if we do act it is either a cry for help or a reaction to the fear we are feeling. Whether the fear is real or imagined doesn't matter to us; it's still overwhelming. When I'm afraid I crawl into a hole and wrap myself in my blankets and pretend I don't exist.

I have to confess I get angry when people take their own fears out on those of us with mental health difficulties. I also get angry when the mental health system lets me down and makes things worse. These days I'm trying to channel that anger into a productive force to challenge the status quo—I want to see things change, because I know my label will remain and will likely cause more severe problems down the line.

The attack that caused my impaired vision

One incident was very serious for me because it caused my impaired vision. But the reason I want to share it with you is because it shows how people with mental health difficulties are still treated.

At the time of the incident I was very unwell and in the middle of a severe psychotic period. I was a resident in a 24-hour-staffed residential rehabilitation unit, but I walked out because I wanted to commit suicide by jumping off Trent Bridge. To get there I had to walk through housing estates and I admit I must have looked odd in my pyjamas and coat with no shoes or socks.

When I stopped for a rest because I was getting panic attacks, some boys called to me. I remember hearing one of them say, 'I want to report a dead body, not a live body'. Then I felt something hit the back of my head, and when I woke up I saw the shadow of a policeman.

I could hardly see a thing at that point. I don't know if it was the shock or the blow on the head but I felt dizzy and sick and I was still hearing voices.

When the ambulance arrived they were more concerned to assess me for my mental health than my injuries. I told them I'd been attacked. My ribs hurt and I came up in bruises a few days later so I assumed that had happened while I was unconscious. But they were more concerned about the state of my mind than my body.

Now I accept that I must have looked bizarre, but that incident led to the loss of some of my vision, so although I did have serious mental health problems I should have received the same care for the physical attack as anyone else.

Diary: June 2004

"I have been undertaking a course on training for trainers. Hopefully this will lead to better training for staff in the National Health Service, giving them some insight into mental health problems from a service user perspective."

I have an ambition to challenge people's perceptions about mental ill-health and recovery. I don't want others to receive the poor service I had and if I can use my experience to highlight constructive areas of change, I will. Through talking to clients and staff and the people I meet, I am hopeful that attitudes will start to change, and even if I can change only one person's perspective, I will be happy.

The stigma and the discrimination that are out there are appalling, to say the least, and that includes workers in the service who are supposed to help. Things are slowly changing but are just that: *slow*. The same nurses who worked in the asylums and institutions are still working and unfortunately little has changed in their authoritarian ways.

We might have care in the community but I am still isolated from the real world. I am known as a mental health service user *before anything else*.

People don't see me as capable, intelligent, caring and loving, someone with potential—no—they see me as a service user, incapable in all ways, needing to be doped to the eyeballs. I've also been regarded as the scum that you wipe off your shoes and, of course, seen as potentially dangerous, although I have never hurt a fly! Well, perhaps a fly, but nothing else.

I was filled with potential and ambition at 18. Like many at my age I had started university to become a teacher and then in the third year I crashed. Because of my current problems I feel as if I'm treated as being incapable of achieving anything ever again, doomed to be a service user for the rest of my life.

I absolutely do not believe this. I may never be 100% well, but I am a worthwhile human being with a lot to give to society.

Three ways to help

1. When you meet someone with a mental health problem, try not to fit them into a 'category'.

2. Even if someone seems to be having difficulties, don't assume they are unintelligent. As one person said, "My mental health problems don't rob me of my intelligence; they simply reduce my ability to cope."

3. If you aren't sure how to address them, ask them what they prefer to be called, because first and foremost they are *them*.

Abnormality

What is abnormal?

Edgar Allan Poe wrote: "**Men have called me mad, but the question is not yet settled whether madness is or is not the loftiest intelligence—whether much that is glorious—whether all that is profound—does not spring from disease of thought—from moods of mind exalted at the expense of the general intellect.**"

Ok, so what is normal? Definition, please! Can you define what is *normal*?

If my life is the same every day, that is normal for me even if it seems odd to you. If I did exactly the same things you did throughout the day and thought about exactly the same things, would that be normal? Of course not, unless, perhaps, you and I were identical twins! Even so, my friend's daughters are identical twins and they certainly have different characters as well.

Perhaps the realisation when I was young that I was different from other people was correct, because we *are* all different.

As human beings we are individuals on one long continuum:

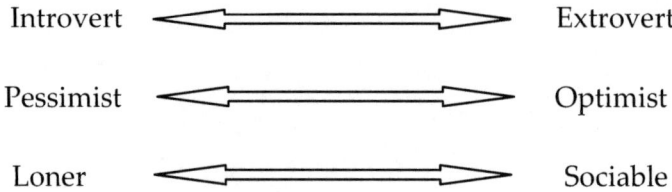

This list could be carried on forever.

In our society, what is normal?

Let's start off with a definition of 'normal' to help us decide what's *ab*normal'.

Normal: "Approximately average in any psychological trait such as intelligence, personality or emotional adjustment"

"Free from any mental disorder, sane"

I know what people in my society think is abnormal and that is anyone not seen to be behaving normally for the situation they are in, in that society, at that time.

If I was dancing and singing in the street, would that be normal behaviour? It would be normal if it was a part of a celebration or festival, but not if it was me alone in the city centre.

Even then, if I was Spanish and more extroverted, would I be abnormal in that situation even if I *were* dancing alone?

We cannot define what normal behaviour is without understanding the context of the person and their behaviour. It is more about what is acceptable behaviour for that time and place. What is acceptable in one society might not be acceptable in another.

So what is abnormal?

A study entitled *"On being sane in insane places"* was carried out by D.L. Rosenhan in 1973, published in Science, 179, 250-58

Rosenhan designed his study to look at how 'abnormal' is categorized—whether we see abnormality in the way we see beauty—whether it's in the eye of the beholder.

The study was constructed by asking eight clinically sane people to gain admittance into acute psychiatric wards with the intent of studying and researching the culture on the wards. They claimed beforehand that they heard words that others could not, eg 'thud'. Otherwise they behaved as they usually would. All but one were admitted and given a diagnosis of schizophrenia. As soon as they were admitted they said they no longer heard these words and they behaved as usual. Their subsequent behaviour was then observed—with that diagnosis in mind—so when on the wards they sat down and wrote, the act of writing was interpreted *through the diagnosis* instead of being seen as simply writing. The observed mood swings (which we all suffer from), were interpreted not merely as the person being tired, or hungry or bored or frightened, but as an integral part of the diagnosis given. Every behaviour trait was pathologised. This was also my experience on the acute ward. Similar studies have been carried out with very similar results.

If you're a psychiatrist you have a stamp of approval to judge what is normal or, more to the point, what is abnormal, and what is therefore classed as a mental health disorder. Who is best placed to make this judgment? Is it the psychiatrist who sees me for only ten minutes every couple of months (if I am lucky), or is it the people who know me best—including myself?

If my beliefs are not the same as the psychiatrist's *opinion* (there are no simple ways of arriving at a diagnosis and psychiatrists often disagree with each other), should I get a diagnostic label just for that?

Well, I did. I disagreed with my psychiatrist and that was therefore seen as *abnormal* and part of a disorder that needed to be treated and kept under control. It was only after speaking to other like-minded people who saw me as an ordinary human being with potential that I realized I wasn't as MAD as I had been led to believe!

I am white, middle-class and female, brought up in a family in a small village in the United Kingdom and I certainly consider myself to have a number of problems that are abnormal: or are they?

You *could* say that they are completely normal reactions to life events; that my ways of coping are just normal ways of coping that anyone would adopt if given the right circumstances.

It's often said of abused children that they accept their upbringing as 'normal' because it is what they are familiar with; they know no other way.

Reasonable people are abnormal?

I heard someone say once that reasonable people don't change the world. That's because they accept what is and don't do anything to alter it.

When you look at many of the things that we've achieved as humans, they've happened because of someone's obsession; someone with a conviction that something can be improved, done more quickly, more easily, more efficiently.

> ➤ The four minute mile happened because one man believed it possible and set out to achieve it.

➢ Electricity happened because Edison was prepared to be called a failure when he tried ten thousand ways to make it work.

➢ Marconi was regarded as obsessed in his native Italy and had to travel to England to gain acceptance of his ideas about wireless telegraphy

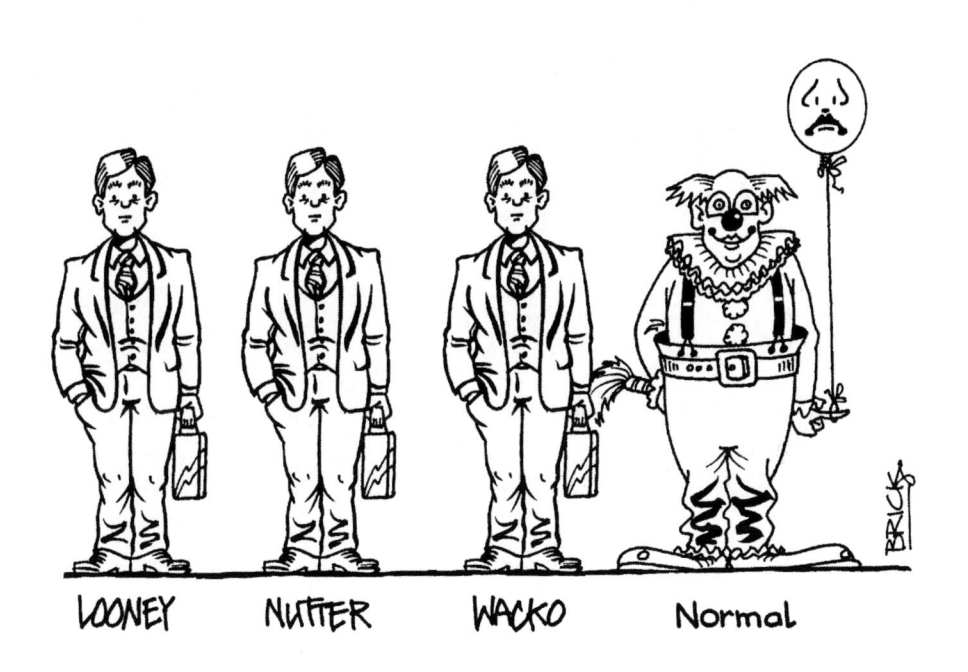

LOONEY   NUTTER   WACKO   Normal

Creativity and mental illness

Ben Okri: "The most authentic thing about us is our capacity to create, to overcome, to endure, to transform, to love and to be greater than our sufferings."

There may be a link between mental illness and creativity, which would explain why some of the greatest and most ground-breaking composers of classical music are believed to have had mental health problems. How do we know? Through evidence such as family history of mental disorder; incarceration in the then 'insane asylums'; vivid descriptions of their emotional experiences in letters to intimates; and of course, in the music itself.

Beethoven, who once contemplated suicide, was described by his contemporaries as heavy-drinking and violent-tempered.

Berlioz was afflicted by black depressions and tried to kill himself.

Bruckner had a nervous breakdown and was hospitalized for mental illness.

Tchaikovsky was manic-depressive and is thought by some to have committed suicide.

Rachmaninoff was afflicted with deep depressions and dedicated his Second Piano Concerto to his psychiatrist.

We only have to look at the lives of some of our most famous artists, poets, playwrights and actors to see that creativity and artistry often go hand in hand with deep inner turmoil.

Try to imagine a world without the ability to hallucinate

('imagine': ability to form images and ideas in the mind, especially of things never seen or never experienced directly', Bloomsbury Concise English Dictionary.)

- Engineers do it all the time when they mentally create a bridge or a road where none may exist now

- Mathematicians and physicists spend their time thinking about things that they'll never see but are convinced underpin all of life

- Artists and musicians see and hear life in new ways that over time the rest of us accept as being 'the norm'

- Some cultures actually induce a hallucinatory state of mind through the use of herbs and other substances to attain an expanded level of awareness

Three ways to help

1. Try to understand that what you see as a negative aspect of a person's illness may be seen by them as a positive.

2. Remember that a recent buzz phrase in the world of business and commerce has been 'think outside the box', to improve creative thinking. The person with mental health difficulties may see things from outside the box *all the time*.

3. We are all too quick to judge. Take time to find out and imagine what it is like from that person's perspective.

Abuse

Defining abuse is complex and rests on many factors. The term 'abuse' can be widely interpreted.

However, abuse is defined in the *Department of Health No Secrets* guidance as the 'violation of an individual's human and civil rights by any other person or persons'.

Abuse may happen as the result of deliberate intent, negligence or ignorance.

Why is it so difficult for people to discuss their abuse?

One of the key factors in any abuse is the control the abuser exerts over the adult or child they are abusing.

If an adult abuses a child then the child will often assume the adult is right, which sets the control mechanism in place. When that is reinforced with verbal or physical threats then the child is doubly cut off and isolated from any possibility of asking for help.

Just as with adults who feel that their friends and family should be able to see they are hurting and do something to help, so a child assumes that other adults around would know if it was wrong and intervene. When that doesn't happen the onus is on the child to act, which for most children is impossible.

Such control, once established, is soon reinforced by the abuser and becomes the norm for the abused person.

In consequence, the ability to speak out, even as an adult, in bullying and abusive situations, becomes difficult. It is well documented that adults abused as children are more vulnerable to problems such as bullying, mental health difficulties and abuse.

'Is it my imagination this is happening?'
'Have I attracted the behaviour by what I did?'
'Will it get worse if I report it to someone?'
'What if my abuser finds out and comes after me?'

If the abuser is in some position of authority over the abused person, then avenues of help are closed off. For example, in the case of mental health service users, who is more likely to be believed, the staff on an acute ward, or the service user?

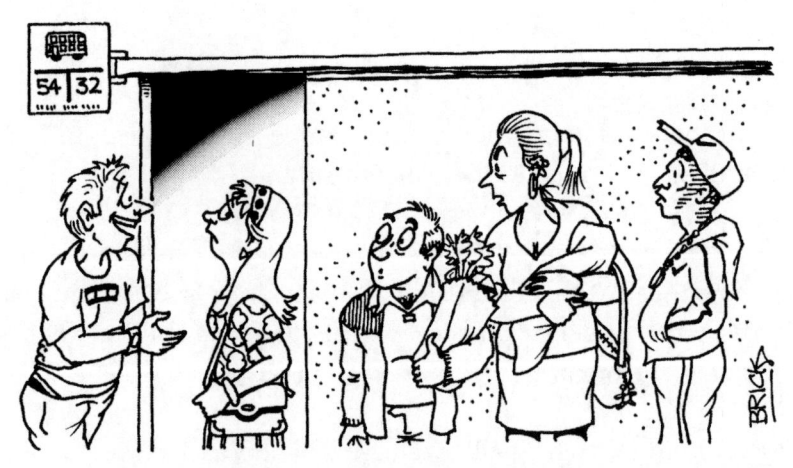

"So listen, I'm here for you anytime you want to talk about being a victim of child abuse..."

Diary: 2005

"I was only five when my life changed. I don't know how to describe it.

As a child I don't remember much about the abuse itself. I blocked it out—I mean really blocked it out. People think you must remember something, but I didn't. I just know things had changed, I knew I'd been naughty and I knew I wasn't supposed to say anything. But I didn't know what about. It was gone: but it wasn't gone.

I still don't know who abused me as a child. But I do have flashbacks and some of them are horrific and I shall never get used to them. One flashback was of manure being stuffed into my mouth and my hand scrabbling on the side of the stable I was in. I was on the top of a hay bale and I do remember that hand. It was rough and gruff. Later it made sense because there were some men I just didn't get on with but didn't know why. Unconsciously I was taking it out on them because they reminded me of the person who'd abused me.

I remember his hands—strong, demanding, controlling, making me stiff as a board so he could do what he wanted with me. It has taken me years to piece together these bits of memory and to even talk about it with anyone. I was told not to utter a word and not a single word did I speak about it till I was nearly twenty years of age.

I went from thinking everybody was lovely, that the world was fantastic, and feeling very safe and content, to being scared. Being scared of people included my so-called friends at school, who bullied me.

I had one friend and that was my dog. She was wonderful. Her name was Flip and I used to walk her and listen to music. That was my route to escape.

The problem was that the voices I began to hear after that abuse comforted me as well as distressed me. So I grew up in a world where the hallucinations, the voices I was experiencing, were more real than real people in life."

How do you begin to unravel a truth about an abuse?

My parents could not understand the endless screaming and tantrums I had as soon as I returned from school that day and quite a number of days after that. I was only five, too young to try and explain, too young to understand and too young for something like this to happen.

Diary: January 2004

"I saw my psychologist today. We discussed lots of things including my past abuse. I found it difficult to talk about the tactile hallucinations. I talked about how I saw male workers not as sexual beings and more as father figures. I talked about how I found female workers more difficult and I realised this linked with the difficulties I had with my Mum.

I began talking about how difficult I found relationships and any tactile contact. I haven't hugged my Mum since I was around four or five and find any tactile contact makes me feel vile and disgusting. I stiffen like a board when someone brushes past me. He challenged me that, like my anxiety and agoraphobia, it will spiral if I don't do it i.e. touch people, and the more I do it the easier it will get. So my task this week is to try tactile contact and to report back how it felt."

Diary: May 2004

"In the sessions we have been talking about the abuse I suffered as a small child and also at 15 years of age. I remember all about the abuse at 15 but I recall very little from when I was five. It was only in this last session that I talked in more depth about the abuse. I wanted to cry but found I was blocking it. That's half my problem; I block my emotions, but they find other ways of coming out either as hallucinations or as self-harm. I found it awkward to talk about it and the psychologist also admitted he found it hard.

He found it hard to imagine what it must be like for a woman to be treated the way I had been treated. And though he could try to empathise, it was *something he hadn't experienced for himself.*

After the abuse had happened I couldn't cope. It was then that I realised that something had happened when I was little as the rush of feelings that I had experienced when I was little had come back again after the later abuse.

Oh those feelings of powerlessness, guilt, disgust, dirt. No matter how much I washed I could not rid myself of the dirt. Was it my fault that he raped me? Did I lead him on? Why me? It was these questions that I had been raising with the psychologist now.

I still don't have answers. He suggested that I might have been intrigued by his advances and half of me curious. No, I was **SCARED**; my body froze. I knew he would do it and nothing I did could prevent it. I tried to push him away but I couldn't say "No!" I didn't feel I had any power to say anything. I was frightened my parents would return from the walk and how they would react.

When it was over I had a bath and scrubbed and scrubbed. He left. My parents returned and I was going to tell them; they would probably know something was wrong anyway. They didn't. They were happy. I tried to behave normally—well, normally for me. I had been strange and distant now for years. I spent a lot of time in my room. Now all I wanted was to be alone, to hide from the world; this was the only way I felt safe."

Three ways to help
if you think someone has been abused:

1. Respect their privacy. Don't force them to tell you anything until they are ready.

2. Listen without comment, without judgement, without trying to make it right for them.

3. When you're talking to them make sure they are in an environment that represents safety to them.

Exclusion or Isolation:

a state of feeling disliked or alone

Discrimination

Discrimination is "treatment or consideration of, or making a distinction in favour of or against, a person or thing based on the group, class, or category to which that person or thing belongs rather than on individual merit: *racial and religious intolerance and discrimination.*"

To begin with I called this section *Discrimination* because it is common among those of us who have mental health problems. But then I thought that calling it by this name wouldn't get across properly the *feelings* that the discrimination leads to. These for me have been feelings of *exclusion* and *isolation*.

I accept that there are many types of discrimination and maybe you feel that you have suffered as well. It seems as if there are as many ways of being excluded as there are people.

The Blue Eyes Experiment

In the 1960s an elementary school teacher in Iowa, Jane Elliott, carried out an experiment with her class. She divided the class into two groups: brown eyes and blue eyes. Anyone with another eye colour was an outsider and didn't take part. She gave the brown-eyed children preferential treatment, withdrew privileges from the blue eyed and made them wear identifying strips of cloth.

Within 30 minutes previously confident, blue-eyed children regressed to being timid and uncertain. Brown-eyed children with dyslexia suddenly spelled words Elliott knew they'd never been able to spell before.

To her horror Elliott discovered that you can create discrimination. As long as some people seem weaker than others then the stronger will take advantage of that.

I was discriminated against when I was living at the residential unit. There were some lads who called me *'psycho'* and *'nutter'*. I've got friends who've had 'psycho' and 'nutter' written on their walls at Halloween.

I have other friends who have had egg and flour thrown at their windows. And I know other people who've attended my support group who can't go out into their own neighbourhood through fear of what people might say or do to them.

That is really hard. I'm very lucky because I now live in a more rural setting where people take the time to get to know you. And because they take the time to get to know you first, when you mention you have mental health problems they're more than likely to be intrigued and more inclined to accept you as who you are, rather than judge you by a label.

Diary: July 2004
"I tried in the week to catch the bus to the nearest town, like my psychologist suggested last week. I got to the bus stop, had a panic attack and hid behind the pub till I calmed down. Then I burst into tears. I'm not sure of the name of the lady who brought me back home, but it was kind of her.

Unfortunately, I am now preoccupied with thoughts about what people are saying about me and haven't been able to open my curtains since. I hear them talking outside and although I know it is probably my paranoia, it makes me think 'are they talking about me?'
I feel I let myself and my Gran down. I was catching the bus to get to my Gran so she had company for the day."

When I lived in the inner city, if I was doing odd things people stared at me and called me names, and that's really not good.

I understand that when people with mental health problems do unusual things, like talking to themselves in the street or wandering about half-dressed, it can seem frightening. But *they* are the ones in a state of terror, not the onlooker. If people feel that they can't do anything, they should at least not make the situation worse for the sufferer.

I wish I had something physically wrong with me instead of having a mental health difficulty, because then people could actually see there was something wrong. If I had a broken leg they'd see it as an obvious problem and respond appropriately. But with a mental health problem there's often nothing to see on the outside. Take today, for example; I'm waffling and umming and aahing on the tape, writing sections for the book. I've been hearing voices all morning and it's the first period of quiet I've had, so I thought I'd record the tape. But—people can't see that. They can't see the fact that hearing voices or experiencing depression or delusions is exhausting. It's exhausting to fight and it's exhausting to live with.

What follows is how the effects of medication contribute to the feelings of isolation.

Medication should be for most people the last port of call rather than the first. Medication doped me up so much I could no longer think and I could no longer walk properly. I couldn't even talk properly and I was drooling. The walking was like walking in different directions at the same time and your feet and your legs feel so heavy and weighted down that you have no choice but to walk 'funny'. You try not to but you do. And then there's all the agitation and the shaking. Even on the small amount of medication I'm on now, my joints ache from head to toe.

Every single joint aches and I suppose it's like having rheumatism but without actually having rheumatism. It's horrible; you just can't get comfortable anywhere you sit. And when I used to shake (I still shake a little bit now at times), it looks as if you've got Parkinson's disease. I am told the long-term effect of the medication is called Parkinsonism, which basically means experiencing the same side-effects as if you have Parkinson's, and it comes from taking antipsychotics. There is a probability, too, that it can become permanent.

All this contributes to your looking strange, and as a consequence you feel more excluded because you *do* look strange. It's not necessarily because of the mental health difficulties, it's the side-effects of the medication—the weight gain, the shakiness, the way you walk, the drooling. It's **so hard**.

Half my problem is that I care too much about what other people think about what I do. For example, I get paranoid that my bin should go out on time on bin day and be brought back as soon as the bin men have been, so as not to upset the neighbours. When I self-harmed I worried about what others would say about the wounds on my arms.

All these things make my life more isolated than it was before, making my self-esteem and self-worth plummet to zero again. It has taken me a long long time to realise that I am a *valuable human being*.

Three ways to help

1. Be aware of anyone around you who is withdrawing from their usual ways of communication.

2. Be aware of any atmosphere of harassment or bullying where you work, or where you enjoy social activities.

3. Make positive statements of concern within a safe environment for the person.

Agoraphobia

Unexplained fear of open spaces

My fear of leaving a safe place

Agoraphobia is a horrible, debilitating symptom of mental health distress and to me it meant I couldn't go to the shops or even take the bin out to the front gate. At the thought of doing those things I would get a horrible ache in my chest that would build up and up throughout the whole of my body.

When I first started getting chest pains I thought I was having a heart attack or angina, but I wasn't. What I was experiencing were panic attacks, and the chest pain was linked to the anxiety. Full-blown panic attacks are horrendous—you think that you are dying. No matter how many times you are told that you are not, it still feels as if you are. You can't catch your breath and the more you try to breathe the worse the anxiety builds up. I was agoraphobic for nearly 8 years and during this time I rarely ventured from the house. When I did go out I asked my parents to stay close by, and sometimes I had one each side of me. The more I didn't leave the house, the more I didn't want to leave the house and the cycle of anxiety and panic spiralled out of control. Even when I became a recluse in my bedroom, the anxiety never went away. I didn't even find peace when I was asleep as the nightmares continually haunted me.

So how did I overcome my fear of going out? The *answer* was simple, but in fact it was a slow and painful recovery. I had to battle my fear of meeting people, communicating and socialising again. I had to take it step by step, inching forward, challenging myself every day to a new task. At first it was just standing at the open door, and then it was slowly venturing further and further down the path towards the gate. Every time I ventured further the anxiety would raise its head again and again. But I knew that I had to face my anxiety. Eventually, and I am talking *years*, I was finally able to go out, but even now on some days I find it hard to face leaving the house.

I know I still have to battle with my anxiety every day. But I do *not* want to become a recluse again.

Catching buses was my hardest challenge to overcome. To some people catching a bus is a simple and uncomplicated task, but for me it is still an ordeal. I often have to get off the bus before my stop and then catch the next bus to continue my journey. This isn't helped by the fact that I hear voices on the bus from people who are sitting nearby. I know they aren't really talking about me, but it is unnerving and upsetting that I think they are. It has taken me years—it seems more like a lifetime—to accept that this anxiety will never fully go away.

I have now accepted more of myself, and through overcoming agoraphobia I have realised that I have more strength than I could ever have imagined. If you had asked me ten years ago whether I could go through all that I have been through, then I would definitely have said, "No way!" I suppose I have learned something incredible about myself.

I now catch buses and trains and planes, and although I am not fully at ease, at least I can do it, which is something I thought I would never be able to achieve

Depression

When does 'feeling down' become depression?

Rollo May: **"Depression is the inability to construct a future."**

About 2 in 3 adults in the UK suffer depression during their lives. Serious episodes occur in about 1 in 4 women and 1 in 10 men. In psychiatric terms, depression is defined as an event so severe as to be considered abnormal, either because of no obvious environmental causes, or because the reaction to unfortunate life circumstances is more intense or prolonged than would generally be expected.

What causes depression?

Depression can stem from many life-events such as bereavement, stress or bullying in the workplace, relationship problems or accidents.

Any event that causes you to feel unable to cope, for whatever reason, can lead to depression. For some people such events can spiral them into a cycle of low self-esteem and inability to cope, and the resultant depression deepens.

Women are more prone to depression than men, possibly because of hormonal swings that become extreme. Men, however, can suffer more deeply because they don't want to admit they can't cope. A common reaction is to bottle up all feelings, so that help from family or friends is brushed off, even if the person is screaming inside for help.

Psychiatrists use a manual (DSM 4 or ICD 10) to decide on your diagnosis. They will look at your symptoms and decide if you have enough symptoms to fulfil the requirements for that diagnosis.

Official medical definition of clinical depression:

A person can be diagnosed as suffering from clinical depression if:

(1) Five (or more) of the following symptoms have been present during the same 2-week period and represent a change from previous functioning, and at least one of the symptoms is either number i) (depressed mood) or number ii) (loss of interest or pleasure):
- Depressed mood most of the day and nearly every day, as indicated by either subjective report (e.g. feels sad or empty) or observation made by others (e.g. appears tearful);
  Note: in children and adolescents it can be 'seems irritable';
- Markedly diminished interest or pleasure in all, or almost all, activities most of the day, nearly every day (as indicated by either subjective account or observation made by others);
- Significant weight loss when not dieting, or weight gain (e.g., a change of more than 5% of body weight in a month), or decrease or increase in appetite nearly every day;
  Note: in children, failure to make expected weight gains;
- Insomnia or hypersomnia nearly every day;
- Psychomotor agitation or retardation nearly every day (observable by others, not merely subjective feelings of restlessness or being slowed down);
- Fatigue or loss of energy nearly every day;

- Feelings of worthlessness or excessive or inappropriate guilt (which may be delusional) nearly every day (not merely self-reproach or guilt about being sick);
- Diminished ability to think or concentrate, or indecisiveness, nearly every day (either by subjective account or as observed by others);
- Recurrent thoughts of death (not just fear of dying);
- recurrent suicidal ideation but without a specific plan, or suicide attempt, or specific plan for committing suicide.

(2) The symptoms do not meet the criteria for a Mixed Episode

(3) The symptoms cause clinically significant distress or impairment in social, occupational, or other important areas of functioning

(4) The symptoms are not due to the direct physiological effects of a substance (e.g. a drug of abuse, a medication) or a general medical condition (e.g., hypothyroidism)

(5) The symptoms are not better accounted for by bereavement, i.e. the loss of a loved one; or the symptoms persist for longer than two months or are characterized by marked functional impairment; morbid preoccupation with worthlessness; suicidal ideation; psychotic symptoms; or psychomotor retardation

Unfortunately, the problem with this set of criteria is that sometimes symptoms are present but alongside others, or they are present as a result of the side-effects to prescribed drugs. I fit many of the requirements for more than one of the diagnoses as described in the manuals,

but my symptoms do not fit neatly into one diagnosis and they overlap into many others. I do not fit the box they have put me into, and worse, the label I have been given will follow me for life and affects the treatment I can get. I have had eight different diagnoses in the last 15 years, all very different, all affecting how I am treated and what treatment I am offered or able to access.

Diary: August 2004

"I seem to be going in circles all the time. I fight to get better, then I go downhill, crash and hit rock bottom. Then I struggle to climb back up again. It's a long climb.

I want to be happy, have good friends, a husband and a family. I want to be able to cope with the day, be able to feel full of life. I want to feel whole and alive, energetic, have a lust for life: but I don't.

Good news—I went to the hospital to the endocrine clinic and my thyroid levels are back in the mid-normal range. My prolactin too is down. I have had low thyroid for the last eight years but it went undiagnosed as my psychiatrist wouldn't do the blood test I so very much needed. I knew I had a low thyroid as I had all the symptoms that my Mum had when she was younger. I eventually went privately to have the test and it was then they found I had a high prolactin level, low iron and low thyroid.

My body has thought it has been pregnant for the last six years. I even produced milk for all that time, not a nice experience in anybody's book, so I am glad that the tests came back satisfactory. I still feel that I am not on enough thyroxin supplements as I still feel so tired, but this could be down to the antipsychotics that I am taking for the hallucinations.

The theory that taking your meds gets rid of the voices is nonsense! They never go, although the tablets help me cope better with them. The side-

effects, though, are unpleasant, although the one I am on at the moment is better than the others.

The tablets also mean I have lost any sex drive I once had. I still feel stiff and achy and sometimes jittery, but these are still the best tablets I have been on, although they also make me tired, which doesn't help the depression when it hits, and yes, I take medication for that as well and yes, more side-effects!"

Three ways to help

1. If you're suffering from depression, get help. This does not necessarily mean help from the health services as there are many other support networks and organisations out there. Yes, it will take some time, but seeking help may shorten your recovery time and avoid a major crisis.

2. If you're trying to help someone with depression, know there are choices other than drugs. But you can't magic the person's depression away. It may be a long road and you need patience; and *you yourself* also need support and time out.

3. Acknowledge that it may take a variety of strategies to cope over the period of the depression.

Remember, you are not alone

Bulimia

Bulimia is also called Binge-Purge syndrome. Bulimia Nervosa is often associated with Anorexia Nervosa but can be a separate condition.

It is a disturbance in eating behaviour which often affects young women who believe that their healthy body is overweight. Excessive food intake is followed by self-induced vomiting to prevent weight-gain.

Anorexia and bulimia were given great prominence when it was learned that Princess Diana suffered. Current campaigns are trying to address the zero size obsession of many young women which has led to the rising numbers of female sufferers.

In 2008 John Prescott drew attention to his suffering from bulimia in his autobiography. Despite the jokes at his expense, it shows that it isn't only women who suffer.

Whatever causes it in individuals, one of uniting factors is low self-esteem.

Diary: 3rd February 2004
"I talked about my weight and how I saw myself as being humungous. I mentioned that I had always been told that I was fat and needed to lose

weight. When I was only 14 I went to WeightWatchers with my Dad. I thought that I was huge then, but I wasn't. When I look back at the photos I wasn't huge at all; I was a normal teenager. I know that my low thyroid had already started as all the signs were there. I lost the weight but then I put it all straight back, with extra pounds on top.

I know I comfort-binge. It's more than a habit; it's a way of coping. I still binge and purge. I hate myself and what I have done to myself and what I still do, including the cutting and other self-harm.

I talk about my bingeing and purging. My psychologist said that we could come to some agreement—perhaps decide only to binge on alternate days and that's its ok to binge every other day and not to feel bad about it. I said that with the work coming up next week in Wales I didn't think I could keep to that. So we decided it was something for the future.

I told him how frightened I was about next week, so the conversation turned to coping strategies. I feel stressed and I know it's going to be hard, physically and emotionally.

We also talked about failure. He wants me to experience it. I don't. I know I am not good at failing. I take it as a reflection on myself. I want to do things at my best and feel that as long as I have done my best that's all I can do, and that I should feel good. But if I don't do my best then that is wrong and I would feel disheartened with myself. I must talk this through with him next time I see him."

Diary: Friday 7th May 2004

"I have just had my dinner followed by a whole cheesecake. I have had my eye on the cheesecake for the last day and a half; it stared at me every time I went in the freezer. I feel bad because I promised myself that I would leave it alone.

I have now emptied my stomach and feel very depressed and angry with myself for doing it in the first place. My Gran always used to give me biscuits and cakes but my Dad didn't think it was a good idea to be fed whole packets of biscuits. It became something naughty and it still feels the same way. It feels now as if I am a small child who has done something wrong.

I wasn't big as a child but I was always treated as big by other children and I thought I needed to lose weight. When I started WeightWatchers at 14 I had to be escorted by my Dad as I was too young to go on my own. I lost the weight then piled it all back on, and more. This was the start of my yo-yo dieting.

Eventually this led to extremes of bingeing and purging. My teeth used to be strong but now they are sensitive and brittle. I get constant heartburn and sometimes bring up blood.

I have already admitted to my psychologist that perhaps I actually subconsciously want to stay fat so I don't attract attention from men."

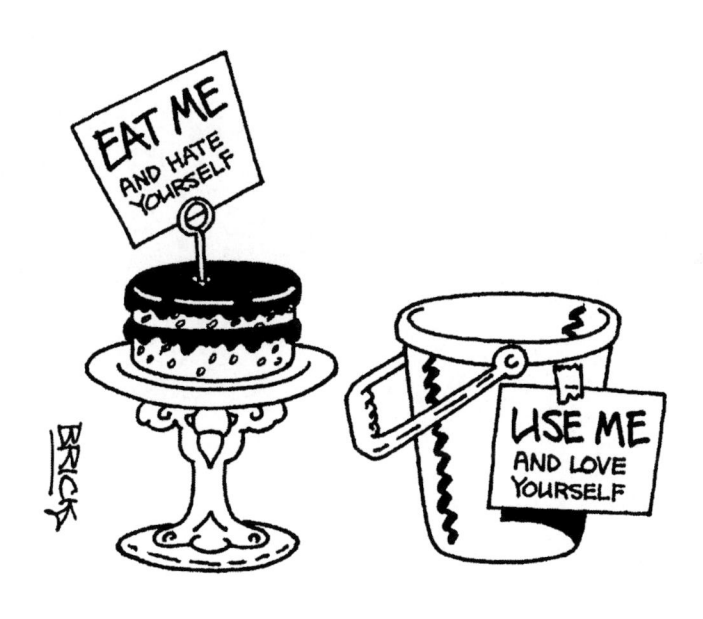

Three ways to help

1. Let them make their own choices. Putting pressure on them doesn't help, even if they know you mean well. Bulimia is a coping strategy and can't simply be switched off.

2. Make sure they know you still love them. Bulimia sufferers often feel isolated because of how they view food and the reasons for developing this way of coping need time to be addressed.

3. Help them to find ways of dealing with bulimia, but realise that their chosen way may not be what you expect.

Self-harm

Self-injury (SI) or self-harm (SH) is deliberate injury inflicted by a person upon his or her own body without suicidal intent.

These acts may be aimed at relieving otherwise unbearable emotions, sensations of unreality and numbness. It is often associated with mental traits such as low self-esteem or perfectionism. Non-fatal self-harm is common in young people worldwide and this term is now increasingly used to describe any non-fatal acts of deliberate self-harm, no matter what the intention is.

"A significant proportion of the mental health workload in A&E in the UK is related to self-harm, which is one of the top 5 causes of acute medical admissions for both men and women." (*National Framework p33*)

"It is essential that people who have self-harmed receive a specialist psychosocial assessment before discharge, preferably performed by a mental health nurse or other professional who knows local services and can arrange speedy follow-up and appropriate support."(*National Framework p33*)

I know someone who self-harms who, when he went to A & E to get help, not only did he *not* see a mental health nurse or receive any support whatsoever, he was accused of being a time-waster. Because of this experience he did not access any further much-needed help. With that kind of reception, those of us who self-harm in this way are unlikely to want to admit it to others. It also further reduces any self-esteem and increases the likelihood of needing to continue to self-harm.

We all self-harm

You may regard this heading as a provocative statement but we all have our own ways of 'treating' ourselves or dealing with those stressful times that, when taken to extremes, can harm us. What is *your* way of letting off steam when the pressures build up inside you?

Do you express your frustration by shouting at other drivers on the road?

Do you have just one glass of wine then another, then another at the end of the day?

Do you smoke because it 'helps you relax'?

Do you stay away from your family in the evening because you can't stand the noise of the kids or the nagging of your partner?

The emphasis placed on the rise of binge-drinking, drug taking and eating disorders show that there are many ways of self-harming. Equating those issues with hallucinations, delusions or cutting oneself may seem simplistic. But what one person can cope with long-term, such as a high level of alcohol in the system, can for another person quickly lead to severe problems.

Alcohol is more socially acceptable than drug taking. Some forms of drug taking are more acceptable than the 'nutter' who stands in the street shouting at an unseen person. Acceptable behaviour, as I've already indicated, can depend upon context.

Diary: 1st May 2004

"In the first year of university I tried to make friends but I was paranoid and distant. I started drinking and didn't stop. I took an overdose and landed in Casualty. I asked for help from the GP as I knew I needed help, but the help didn't come. I wonder now whether, if I had had the help I needed then, I would be here now, eight years down the line, still struggling to rebuild my life . . .

My second year of university was further away, in Hull. I spent every weekend coming back home to my safe haven. It was only in the last term that I decided to spend my weekends in the Yorkshire Dales, sometimes paragliding if the weather was right, sometimes just exploring or sleeping."

Sleeping is something I did a lot and still do. I could and still can fall asleep anywhere. I fall asleep if stressed, and I don't mean pretend sleep—it's real, gone sleep. It was out of my control.

When a friend took me to a night club for the first time I fell asleep in a corner, not drunk but completely gone. I even got kicked out once because a bouncer thought I was drunk when I was actually stone-cold sober. I drank heavily through most of that time, even to the point of drinking in the mornings to overcome the inevitable hangover and get through the day.

It was in Hull that my panic attacks started. I thought it was asthma and even went to the GP about it. I started to avoid the places where I had panic attacks—it was usually where there were people.

I went to Nigeria in the summer to teach in a summer school. This was another big mistake.

The panic attacks continued to spiral out of control until during the third year I started to self-harm by cutting myself, just so I could cope.

The self-harm was a way of releasing the stress. It was powerful and addictive.

I would hit my head, too, but it was only when I threw myself down a flight of stairs that my parents knew something was wrong. I had hidden it successfully for a very long time. I started to see a psychiatrist and he prescribed antidepressants.

By now I had withdrawn completely, rarely going out into the world and sometimes being so isolated that I didn't even leave my room, and in the end I didn't even leave my bed. Finally in the March of my third year of university I reluctantly left. My whole world crashed and I landed in hospital.

Three ways to help

1. It may be difficult, but try not to show disgust at the self-harm. That will result in the person who self-harms putting themselves at a distance from you. Remember, self-harm is their main way of coping and surviving.

2. Ask them what you can do to help. It may be that they want you to listen. That takes time and patience when all you want to do is rush off and 'solve' the situation. You need to go at their pace.

3. Don't give them ultimatums. That will only add to the pressure and stress they already feel.

Suicide

Arthur Schopenhauer: "*They tell us that suicide is the greatest piece of cowardice, that suicide is wrong, when it is quite obvious that there is nothing in the world to which every man has a more unassailable title than to his own life and person.*"

Judy Collins: "**For many centuries, suicides were treated like criminals by society. That is part of the terrible legacy that has come down into present day society's method of handling suicide recovery. Now we have to fight off the demons that have been hanging around suicide for centuries.**"

Talking about the suicide or attempted suicide of someone you care about can bring up a range of emotions, from anger to frustration; anger at their attempt or success in exiting a situation that concerns you; frustration that you hadn't or couldn't do anything to stop it.

The Samaritans' creed of allowing a suicidal person free will is a difficult concept for many people to accept.

"They should face the music."

"Nothing can be that bad."

"There are always options."

Suicidal persons feel that their choices have narrowed, through circumstance, temperament or loss of control, to such an extent that suicide is the easiest possible way forward.

Imagine you are carrying a large stone up a hill. The ground underneath your feet becomes rougher and rougher. Then the path disappears and each step you take becomes more and more dangerous. You can't go back but you're afraid to go forward.

With each step you climb the stone feels heavier and heavier. You move it from one shoulder to another, trying to balance it so it's safe. By now you think you should have reached the summit but as you peer upwards you realise that it's getting dark.

Now your steps are smaller. All you really want to do is lay this burden down and go to sleep. It isn't that you want to hurl yourself off the edge of the mountain; you just want to let go the stone, lie down and sleep.

My first suicide attempt was in my second year at university when I locked myself in my bedroom and took an overdose of whatever I could find. I don't think I really wanted to die, and not knowing how much medication I needed to succeed, I didn't take enough.

Diary: June 2004

"I made another friend on the ward, called Wayne. He thought he had an IQ of 160; just a bit impossible! You see, he had grandiose thoughts and ideas.

He left before me and I lost touch. Later on I found out he was in the mental health acute ward in hospital. I tried to ring to see if I could visit, but got nowhere. Then one week later I found he had jumped off the multi-storey car park just outside the hospital.

He was the second person I had known well who had jumped from the same place.

'Sitting on a rock watching creation grow'

That phrase was written down by a friend named Maninder one week before he died. He cared for everything and everyone, even the likes of me.

He helped when I was on my first time on the acute ward where I was on special observations—this means a member of staff is close by you constantly, whatever you are doing. I had cut my wrists in the toilet—my second real suicide attempt. Other attempts had been half-hearted cries for help. This time I didn't want to be found, although I was, an hour later. Two weeks later I came off special observations.

My friend Maninder had been rocking endlessly in a chair and asking for help, but the staff just walked by. Half an hour later I could not find him anywhere. I knew he was not supposed to leave the ward as he was on close observations being checked every ten minutes.

Then I found out he too had jumped from the car park. I went to the funeral and cried my heart as he had been a gentle giant to me while I was ill. I didn't even understand the service as it was in a different language, but the loss we all shared.

He had times when he would throw chairs across the room but I knew he needed to let out his frustration and that he would never aim them at me. He even broke a window. I applauded him and said, '"Well, at least the window will be clean now."

The windows in that place were never clean."

Where do you go if you need help when the world is asleep?

"It's half-ten at night and I am tired, yet I can't sleep. That seems to me like a contradiction in terms; I crave a deep sleep yet I know I won't get any—not decent sleep anyway. My head is full, or should I say overflowing, with racing thoughts. It didn't help going to my psychologist

today. He admitted therapy is hard work and that yes, therapy can cause depression. Don't I know it!

I had phoned NHS Direct when I felt like this last week. They were no use. They had no time and when I eventually spoke to a doctor he told me to go to bed. But I couldn't; I was too depressed and suicidal. I drank four cans of lager then rang the Samaritans. Unfortunately the chap I got sounded half asleep and I felt sorry for him so I hung up and eventually I went to bed.

Feeling suicidal, for me, at that time and this, is not about killing myself. No, for me tonight it is the ultimate urge to go into a deep sleep and not wake up: ever.

There is no easy way to commit suicide. If there was an easy way I'd have done it. The knotted pain in the chest is a manifestation of the mental hurt and a deep emptiness, sadness and loneliness.

It doesn't help when at times like this there's no one to call upon. I love my family but they don't help in the right way. Yet do I know what the right way is?

Getting through the night always seems the hardest part—every minute, every hour counted again and again. I try to distract myself by writing my diary and watching innocuous TV. I'll make yet another cup of tea and then the hallucinations will probably take over.

Last week I heard the creatures outside, their feet like claws scurrying across the ground and I feared for my cat still outside. I don't usually see things, only when I'm feeling really bad and that was a bad night. My eyesight isn't good anyway but you don't need to see them to feel them out there.

Eventually the cat came in, as calm as anything, but I was frazzled. At least I have my medication this week."

Diary: 1st April 2005

"I haven't written in my diary for a few weeks. I have been too frightened to pick it up. A lot has been happening in my head.

For a start I got so depressed I took an overdose and was in a coma for two days. All I could think when I woke up was, "SHIT! I am still here." It frightens me to know that a lot of the time I still think that. I took so much Olanzapine (an antipsychotic) and Zopiclone (to treat insomnia) that I SHOULD HAVE died. I could not have swallowed any more than I did.

It was nice, just drifting off. I wasn't scared or upset. I was content with my decision, in one way happy that I had made my mind up at last. It was the right decision . . . and in some ways still is. I knew people would be upset afterwards but they would get over it, eventually. And the pain for me would be over.

I don't want to live my life for everyone else except me. I don't know what I want out of life and if I can't enjoy it and find some fulfilment, is it worth it? Should I spend my life living for others while I am in distress?"

That last suicide attempt was the worst I had had and the nearest that I came to succeeding. Things couldn't get much worse. However, it was also the time that I finally decided things were going to change. And if things were going to change it was *I* who had to change them. It was from that point that I started to turn my life around. No, it is not easy and at times still isn't, even today. It was a very hard decision to make. Did I want to live or die? It was cruel to my parents and those around me if I didn't decide once and for all. If I decided to die I should just get on and do it. If I decided to live I needed to move forward and take control back over my life, face my fears and stamp down on any thoughts of ever again taking my own life. It was the hardest decision of my life and not as simple a choice as you might think.

I decided to live.

It was then that the hard work really started.

Three ways to help

1. If someone tells you they feel suicidal, take them seriously, however lightly they talk about it. They need the response that shows them you have heard what they said.

2. Encourage them to talk. It may be distressing for you but remember, it may the first time they feel able to be open about how they are really feeling and it may well be the first step in the process of their recovery.

3. Don't try to 'make it better' for them. Whatever the situation that has caused the suicidal feelings you cannot simply wave a magic wand. They need active, empathetic listening. There is rarely a 'quick fix'; it all takes time.

Psychosis

A group of conditions that affect the mind and to some extent mean that the person loses contact with reality.

A person may experience unusual or distressing perceptions e.g. hallucinations and delusions, which may be accompanied by a reduced ability to cope with the usual day to day activities and routine. Someone who has these unusual experiences is described as having a psychotic episode.

Official attitudes towards psychosis and its treatment are now changing. The following quotes come from the Executive Summary of a report by the British Psychological Society, Division of Clinical Psychology, published in June 2000. The report is entitled *"Recent advances in understanding mental illness and psychotic experiences"*.

"Psychiatric diagnoses are labels that describe certain types of behaviour. They do not indicate anything about the nature or causes of the experiences.

Any mental health difficulty, including psychosis, can be put on a continuum. It is important to recognize that like all other mental health difficulties anyone can have psychotic experiences given the right circumstances e.g. sleep deprivation, dehydration.

Social circumstances are very important. People from disadvantaged backgrounds, especially young men, seem at greater risk of receiving a diagnosis of schizophrenia. However, although the risks may vary, almost anyone could have psychotic experiences in circumstances of extreme stress.

Social, biological and psychological causes of psychotic experiences are all important, and interact with one another. The body, mind and brain are all interlinked, one affecting the other, and it is very difficult to draw a clear line between biological and psychological factors. The causes of psychotic experiences are complex and one single cause will not be found. Sometimes psychotic experiences can be triggered by something relatively minor, but become a problem as a result of some kind of vicious circle involving the initial situation or a person's reaction to their experience.

Psychotic experiences can sometimes follow major events in someone's life, either negative or positive. Many people who have psychotic experiences have experienced abuse or trauma at some point in their lives. The traditional psychiatric drugs are by far the most common form of help offered to people with psychotic experiences. They can be used for acute psychotic experiences and/or used long-term to try to prevent future problems. They do not help everyone."

Unfortunately, many people, including mental health workers, do not realise there are a variety of ways of coping with psychosis other than medication. The Hearing Voices network (see page 164 for contact details) is a good source of support and advice on all options.

Psychosis usually refers to experiences where the person loses touch with reality.

The types of experiences can include:
- hearing voices when no one is there
- seeing or sensing things others do not
- holding strong beliefs that others in the community do not share (often called delusions), some of which relate to the belief that others are out to harm you (called paranoid delusions)
- experiencing extreme moods e.g. depression/elation or both at the same time

- changes in perception (e.g. seeing colours much more brightly than usual)
- feeling much better or worse about one's self than normal

Some people may also:
- find it hard to concentrate on things
- appear distracted or talk back to the voices
- talk in a way which is hard to follow, for example, quickly moving from topic to topic
- feel withdrawn, listless, apathetic or unmotivated

Within medicine and psychiatry such experiences are viewed as symptoms of a mental illness, e.g. schizophrenia, bipolar-affective disorder, schizo-affective disorder.

It is important to remember that many people who have psychotic experiences are not distressed by them and/or do not come into contact with psychiatric services. 10% to 25% of the normal population have had a hallucination at some point in their life (Slade and Bentall 1988). Psychotic-like experiences are 50 times more prevalent than schizophrenia. Extreme experiences, i.e. sensory or sleep deprivation or dehydration, can lead to paranoia and hallucinations. In some cultures, hallucinations are regarded as spiritual gifts rather than as symptoms of having a mental health difficulty.

A study of 18,000 people in the US revealed between 11% and 13% had experienced hallucinations (TIEN, 1991). Therefore about 10 times as many people have experienced hallucinations as receive a diagnosis.
Two-thirds of people who take medication regularly are likely to experience a recurrence of these psychotic experiences within two years.

The medication can have serious, unwanted effects which for some people can be worse than the original problem. New drugs are not necessarily any more effective. Many people are prescribed doses above recommended levels.

People who use mental health services are themselves at risk of becoming victims of violence. They are also at risk of self-neglect, suicide, abuse of human rights and the damaging consequences of treatments. Most people who have psychotic experiences are not dangerous.

People with psychiatric diagnoses are arguably one of the most socially excluded groups in society. Media accounts give a very biased picture and help to maintain public prejudices."

Extra Diary piece written during the summer of 2006

"The postman is talking through my letter box. He's been at it for days. Every morning I dread the sound of the gate as I don't know what he's going to say today. Sometimes he just whispers, sometimes he is louder, but I can hear every word. He tells me what people have said to him as he has done his rounds, usually something about me or my dog.

This morning he was telling me that my dog whines too much and my neighbour hates my dog. He said he is going to poison the dog next time she goes out so I haven't been able to let her go outside to go to the toilet.

In the end I have had to let her out and have followed her every move, just in case. Inside again I ponder every word that the postman has uttered through the door. I know he probably hasn't, and it's my brain working overtime, but that still doesn't stop me from worrying and wondering. Even if it is just my brain creating him talk, why would my brain think something like it does if it wasn't half true in the first place?

I try to be normal when I see the postman in case he hasn't said the things I have heard. I usually check out with people if they have been talking about me to see if they really have or not. That was okay to do when I was at home with my parents, but when it comes to strangers, would they answer honestly anyway?"

Research carried out in the Netherlands in the 1980s came up with over 30% of the respondents to a radio phone-in happily admitting to hearing voices, thinking it was quite normal and not wanting to get rid of the voices.

Seeking understanding

When you hear voices for the first time you will obviously want to try and make sense of what is happening. You will want to understand where they are coming from and why they are there i.e. you will want *to seek understanding*.

God? The devil? The tv? Aliens? These are all ways of trying to understand and make sense of what is going on. It depends on your previous life experiences as to how you interpret these unusual experiences, and your interpretations can and will change over time. It is often easier to believe that the voices are external to yourself and that they are generated elsewhere. This is because voices can be distressing (although some can also be helpful and supportive). Hallucinations for me (and for many other people I know) usually hit home at a very personal level, targeting your innermost fears, and the things that distress you most are usually the things you find hardest to talk about with anyone.

Changing the way you make sense of the experiences can help you to cope with the distress caused by the voices. The more knowledge you have about the voice-hearing experience and just knowing that you are not alone, can help. Understanding that the voices are originating from the inner me and that they feed on my fears and insecurities and what is happening around me, has also helped, although this understanding has taken me most of my life to achieve. It is important to note here that challenging someone's core beliefs about their voices can be very detrimental to them. Believing that a voice is external to yourself makes the experience feel safer, whereas being told it is coming from you, especially when the voices are derogatory about you or your family, can be a shock and potentially harmful. If it can be helpful to believe the voices are external, who has the right to say different, especially if it is helpful to that person and is causing no harm to anyone else? Personally I don't believe in ghosts, aliens or a god (in the traditionally sense), but that doesn't give me the right to say that some one else cannot. Having a belief is helpful, and for the majority of people believing in a God and life after death gives them security, purpose, meaning and comfort.

In the same way, how someone chooses to interpret their voices is their right, if their explanation helps them, even if others don't share that same explanation. A lot of the distress caused by the voices is down to how you interpret them. If you believe that they have power over you or that something horrible is going to happen because of them then this will naturally cause more distress. If, however, you believe that although they are horrible experiences they have no power and nothing dreadful is going to happen because of them, the distress is minimised. I have had some very distressing voices and still do, but because I have a different understanding about where they are coming from and why they are happening, they do not spiral out of control causing more distress than necessary.

What are *my* voices like?

People who do not experience hearing voices tend to think it must be like the internal voice we all get, but outside your head. This is not so. The voices I have experienced are always clear and human and, although they can be quiet or small, they are very real.

They also all have individual personalities and characters. The male voice, 'him', that I still hear today, that I grew up with, has his own very individual personality and character. He's grumpy and moody, swinging from happy to sad to angry and back again. I can imagine what he would look like in the flesh. He would be middle-aged, have wiry, salt and pepper hair, be stressed with life and have a very short fuse and temper. We have all had people in our lives that we love but sometimes hate and it is this kind of relationship that I have with him (a love/hate relationship) but I wouldn't want to be without him altogether. Other voices I have heard might also be real people in my life. I sometimes hear my friends talk about me in another room, and when I go in to talk to them they will not even be there, they will be upstairs.

How can I explain it better to you?

Imagine you were sitting on a bus full of people. One by one each person spoke to you. Except you're not sure they did.

Each person who 'spoke' to you said something critical. Except you're not sure they did.

And every person who walks past you on that bus makes a horrible comment about you. Except you're not sure they did.

By the time you get off the bus you feel that everyone on that bus hates you. Except you're not sure they do.

The voices I hear come in all sorts of guises. A lot of the time on buses I will hear one person start to talk about me and even mention my name. At the end of the bus journey everyone will have talked about me at some point. For a long time, for this very reason, I could not catch buses or even go out of the house, because it caused me to have panic attacks.

What's real and what's not?

It is hard sometimes to distinguish what is real from what is not real. Are the neighbours really talking over the fence? Is it an hallucination? Or is it real?

Hearing things that others cannot is not limited to just hearing people talk. I sometimes hear a child crying in the walls of the house where I live. I hear noises like bumps, crashes and even music which is clear as a bell, as if it is in the room or just next door. Then of course there are the delusions and the paranoia.

I can usually tell I am starting to become worse if I can no longer distinguish which of my experiences are real and which are not. It becomes even harder when I cannot check out at this time, with someone I trust, what is real and what is not. It is at this point that the hallucinations spiral out of control and the delusions kick in. It is very real and at times very frightening, and also confusing.

When the delusions have set in and I no longer begin to question whether they are real or not, when I believe that they are real, this is the point where I have crashed and need help quickly.

I avoid things from spiralling to this point by the coping strategies I have in place.

It is really hard when I hear other people I know talk about me, and although I can distinguish most of the time when the voices are real or not, it is still hard not to react to what has been said when I next meet them. I know my neighbour in all probability does *not* want to poison my pets, even though I have heard him talk about doing this, and that it is probably an hallucination. However, even though I know this, that uncertainty is bound to show in my face when I chat with him the next day. I might even avoid meeting him in the first place.

I become more isolated because of this sort of behaviour and, together with my fear of telling people of my difficulties because of how they might react, plus my lack of social skills, I find it nearly impossible to make any friends. Even when I do make friends, which are few and far between, it is hard to maintain that friendship. There are times when I cannot use the phone, or go out, or don't want any contact with anyone and so I shut people out. I do this so as to be able to cope, but the knock-on effect is that friends find me hard work and rarely understand, especially when it can last for months at a time.

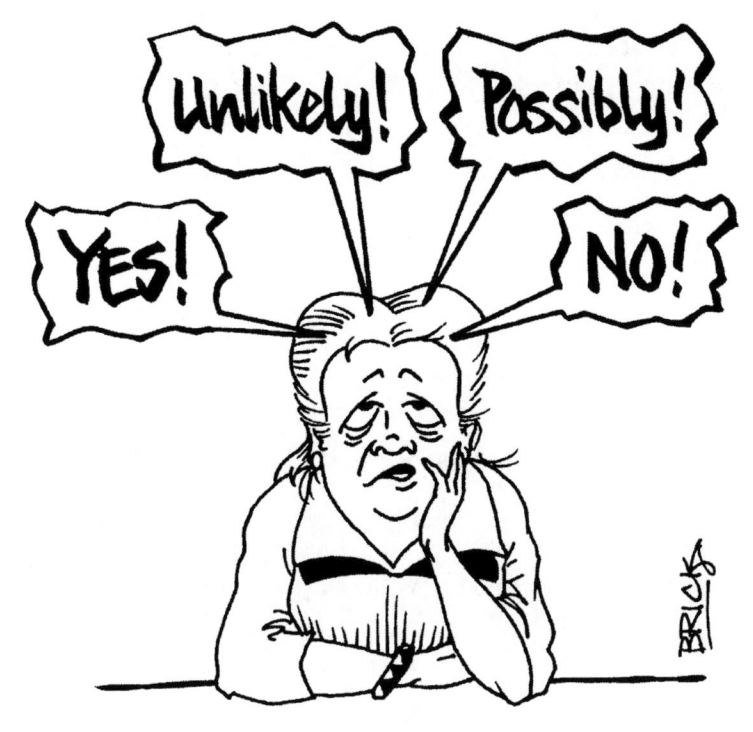

"Just once in my life, can you lot please agree to differ!"

How do I cope with the voices?

My coping strategies might include harmful and even dangerous acts e.g. self-harming by cutting, drinking or eating toxic substances, bingeing and purging etc; but they do help. My strategies also include more positive ways of coping, such as:

- Cleaning
- Hoovering
- Writing
- Listening to music
- Listening to talking books
- Relaxation
- Lavender oil

- Massage
- Acupuncture
- Friends and family
- Checking out with a friend what is real and what is not
- Humming and singing to myself
- Talking back to the voices
- Talking with people I trust about the voices
- Being open about my mental health

However, one of my main strategies is to keep busy and active and includes doing things like writing, teaching, research and working on achieving my degree.

All these latter things must be taken in moderation and at my own pace.

All of the coping mechanisms that I have act as a release for my built-up tension, emotion and thoughts. I never used to be aware that things were building up inside of me. I am now more aware of this than I have ever been and I think this is why I consider myself to be at a certain level of recovery. I can now recognise the signs that I am stressed, down in mood or hyperactive, and then I can do something about it. I have also learnt and now use more of the positive coping strategies I have mentioned, although I sometimes still use the more destructive ones when I really need them.

How do people react to my hearing voices?

Imagine that you were talking to someone you knew and trusted. They said they would introduce you to Becky, who is a trainer in the health service and is completing her degree at the moment.

Before we even met you would have started to build a picture of me. What if your friend then said Becky loves doing yoga and she's writing a book? What would that add to your impression of me?

Then we meet and you might form another impression from my physical appearance. We talk and discover we both like dogs and the same singer. So the conversation is going well and then you ask me what I'm writing about in my book.

I say *"my experiences in the mental health services as a user and the fact that I hear voices"*.

What's your reaction? Is it distaste, misunderstanding, interest or a wish to be as far away from me as possible?

That's how people with hallucinations are often treated (although as I've pointed out earlier, many artists, musicians and writers make use of 'mad' hallucinations to create their work).

Without that disclosure on my part you'd probably have given me the thumbs-up as an intelligent professional with an interesting career. Without the extra information and only the 'hearing voices' label, what would my chances have been to be given the same judgement?

Diary: Monday 29th December 2003

"I define myself as a mental health user and carer. If I was neither, who would I be? That I don't have an answer for because I don't know who I am.

The voices aren't too bad at the moment and I am actually looking forward to Christmas as my Mum has bought me some headphones which hopefully will block out a lot of the voices, temporarily at least."

Diary: 14th January 2004

*"Saw my psychologist today. It left me a lot to think about. We talked about the lack of control that I feel I have and about the 'shoulds'—the things that I feel I **should** do.*

The voices talk a lot about the way the things should be done. The voices from the people on the street are also all about the things I should be doing and about the things I do wrong or think I do wrong.

I think this all stems from my parents as even now there seems to be the right way and the wrong way to do things. I always feel I have to get their permission or approval to do anything. I also feel I can't buy things for myself as they are bound to be wrong."

I may never be without the voices, but one day they won't be as important, as tiresome or as difficult to live with. I have to learn to live for myself rather than for others.

Diary: 3rd February 2004

"The voices are a window into my subconscious, a window I want to shut. They reveal what I really think and what others think of me. I want to be free. I don't want to be able to think. I just want to be able to accept that I am who I am and get on with living a life with meaning. Instead I analyse the meaning of my life, my purpose, my wants, my needs and expectations of myself. I don't want to be me, but I am who I am and I can't change that.

Perhaps there is higher purpose to my life and that this life is just a test and a learning tool and is just the beginning of a long journey, never ending and just starting.

I think too much. It's a habit I ought to break. When I think too much I start to get ill and the voices get worse.

The more I analyse, the more voices I hear. The more voices I hear, the more paranoid I get. The more paranoid I get, the more depressed I become. The more depressed I become, the more isolated and insular and hidden from the world I want to be. It's a cycle I can't seem to break. Not yet, anyway.

I had better get some sleep. I have a long day tomorrow."

Since I wrote that diary entry I've come to accept the voices more and learn how to use them to work through issues they are raising. Just as others use dream analysis for helping them solve problems, I've learned to understand and work with my voices. I've learned the signs that warn me I need to take care. But I've also learned that, listened to carefully, my voices can help me work through problems I'm having.

Ways forward in treatment of psychosis

A recent programme called *Psychosis Revisited* has been run in two centres—West Sussex and Nottingham.

The aim of the two-day workshop was to improve understanding and communication between all those involved in the mental health system; service users, service workers and system administrators.

The importance of involving service users cannot be stressed enough. Their participation was a vital key to helping service workers understand the issues from the inside.

Key issues that were raised at both centres included:
- The importance of shrinking the gap between 'them' and 'us'
- The value of service user views
- The meaning of psychotic experiences
- The importance of encouraging hope
- The value of small talk

Allowing service users to participate in the whole two days rather than simply appearing to give just a segment of the workshop strengthened the value of the experience for all participants.

Those of us who have taken part in these workshops hope that they will become more frequent and a scheduled part of any mental health service staff training.

For me and the psychologists, the way we worked as a team of trainers was refreshing. I do not know whether it was because of the psychologists' view or because of the *Psychosis Revisited* training approach—perhaps both—but it just worked; it all made sense to me and rang true within me. My co-peer trainers were a mix of people and professionals—including those who had experienced mental health distress—psychologists and a mental health nurse. We worked as a team where I was not patronised or labelled but was an equally important contributor. I was and still am an equal.

I wanted to be involved within the whole of the training and not just be rolled out as a subject to be presented in a session, as the manual suggested. This was immediately fine with my colleagues and yes, they were and still are my colleagues. We are on an equal footing as trainers together, all trying to achieve the same aims.

We saw the aims of the *Psychosis Revisited* training as encouraging a change in the attitude and behaviour of mental health staff through education, information and the first hand experience given to them from someone who has used the service. Over the two days, space was given to discuss and reflect on practice.

Although I did not have a label of schizophrenia even though I experienced psychosis, I was not excluded by my co-trainers, although I had expected I would be. My co-trainers did not see the labels people were given; they saw the person and their experience and what they could offer. They did not pretend to know what psychosis was like or that they had the answers, and as I learnt from them they also learnt from me.

I was treated as an equal for the first time in my life. Before this time I had either been treated as a child or a youth, or as mentally ill (i.e. a second-class citizen under the mental health system) by psychiatrists, health workers and nurses. This was a new way of viewing myself; I was now seen as valuable, worthwhile, intelligent and equal, with a lot to offer.

Although they would continue to talk down to me, the mental health services could not take away my new-found sense of self and that I had a right to heard and to be understood. I would not have gained this without being involved in the *Psychosis Revisited* workshop. Many thanks go to the people, my co-trainers and that period of time. It was a very important step in my discovery, working my way towards recovery.

The *Psychosis Revisited* workshops not only helped in my recovery process by making me see myself as someone who is equal, valued and respected, but also helped by the other trainers challenging me as forcefully as I challenged them. The relationship between me and my co-trainers was a true partnership, not tokenistic and not patronising or over-protective.

Three ways to help

1. If you're in a position to involve mental health service users in staff training programmes, please do, because it brings the training to life and is also beneficial to the service user trainer.

2. Try to understand the energy it takes for someone who hears voices to deal with those experiences every day.

3. When you talk to someone with psychotic difficulties, being clear about your intentions can help reassure them.

Section 2

The Mental Health System

The Mental Health Act 1983 is concerned with the reception, care and treatment of mentally disordered patients, the management of their property and other related matters.

Mental *disorder* is defined in the 1983 Mental Health Act as 'mental illness; arrested or incomplete development of mind; psychopathic disorder; any other disorder or disability of mind'. The Act does not define mental *illness*, which is a matter for clinical judgement. (National Framework, p 132)

Difference between mental health difficulties and learning difficulties

Northfield (2004) "What is a learning disability? The World Health Organisation defines learning disabilities as 'a state of arrested or incomplete development of mind'. Somebody with a learning disability is said also to have 'significant impairment of intellectual functioning' and 'significant impairment of adaptive/social functioning'. This means that the person will have difficulties understanding, learning and remembering new things, and in generalising any learning to new situations. Because of these difficulties with learning, the person may have difficulties with a number of social tasks, for example communication, self-care, awareness of health and safety. A final dimension to the definition is that these impairments are present from childhood, not acquired as a result of accident or following the onset of adult illness."

Stewart (2007) "What is mental illness? Mental illness is very common. About one in four people in Britain has this diagnosis, but there is a great deal of controversy about what mental illness is, what causes it, and how people can be helped to recover. People with a mental illness can experience problems in the way they think, feel or behave. This can significantly affect their relationships, their work, and their quality of life."

There are many different types of mental health problems ranging from the more commonly known difficulties such as depression, anxiety, panic attacks and phobias, to the lesser understood difficulties such as OCD (obsessive compulsive disorder), manic depression (bi-polar disorder), schizophrenia and the range of personality disorders.

A mental health difficulty is different in that it could be caused by social stressors, life events, drug problems and a general inability to cope with life.

Mental health problems can affect people from all sections of society although they are more common among people with poor living conditions. Drug or alcohol difficulties are not as common a factor as many people believe.

Mental health problems rarely have just one cause, and even short-term mental health difficulties can be produced by events such as divorce, losing a job or partner, and even moving home.

Hatloy (2008) "The breakdown below gives an overview of what treatment those who experience mental health problems are likely to seek and get:

- around 300 people out of 1,000 will experience mental health problems every year in Britain
- 230 of these will visit a GP
- 102 of these will be diagnosed as having a mental health problem
- 24 of these will be referred to a specialist psychiatric service
- 6 will become inpatients in psychiatric hospitals."

(Source: based on figures from Goldberg, D. & Huxley, P, 1992, *Common mental disorders—a bio-social model*, Routledge)

In September 1999 the government published the *National Service Framework for Mental Health* with the aim of driving up quality and removing the wide and unacceptable variations in provision.

It set standards in five areas:
- **Standard One:** Mental health promotion
- **Standards Two and Three**: Primary care and access to services
- **Standards Four and Five**: Effective services for people with severe mental illness
- **Standard Six:** Caring about carers
- **Standard Seven**: Preventing suicide

I'm quoting from the Framework to show the goals the government has set for the service. If you are new to dealing with the mental health system I hope this will help by outlining the best care that should happen.

The National Service Framework has also laid down three key aims:
- **Safe services**
- **Sound services**
- **Supportive services**

It stated that the standards were challenging and proposed that where parts of the service were providing the best care they should be regarded as milestones for the standard of care to be rolled out across all authorities.

Ways you might end up in the Mental Health Service system

1. Through referral from your GP
2. Through referral from Social Services
3. Through contact with the police
4. Through A&E or NHS Direct

First access to services:

Standard Two:
Any service user who contacts their Primary Health Care team with a common mental health problem should:
- Have their mental health needs identified and assessed
- Be offered effective treatments including referral to specialist services for further assessment, treatment and care if they require it

Standard Three
Any individual with a common mental health problem should:
- Be able to make contact round the clock with the local services necessary to meet their needs, and receive adequate care
- Be able to use *NHS Direct* as it develops, for first-level advice and referral on to specialist helplines or to local services

Standard 4 (NF 41)

All mental health service users on CPA (Care Programme Approach) should:
- receive care which optimises engagement, anticipates or prevents a crisis, and reduces risk
- have a copy of a written care plan which:
    - includes the action to be taken in a crisis by the service user, their carer, and their care co-ordinator
    - advises their GP how they should respond if the service user needs additional help
    - is regularly reviewed by their care co-ordinator
    - be able to access services 24 hours a day, 365 days a year

Diary: Thursday 12th February 2004

"My review: we are supposed to have an assessment every six months, but this time it has been a year. My psychiatrist, community psychiatric nurse (CPN) and a worker from the day centre were there. I was nervous and I am glad I wrote everything down and gave it to my CPN beforehand. I ended up with an increase in my antidepressant Venlafaxine and a decrease in the sedative Lorazapam. Lorazapam is addictive so I had asked for a decrease, which I am sure he was going to suggest anyway. At least it shows I am responsible."

Diary: August 2008

"I still haven't received a copy of my care plan I am supposed to be offered a copy every time it is updated and have the opportunity to be involved and comment on it. This care plan affects how much support I get and in what way I get that support. I don't know what is on the plan, I don't know what support I should be receiving and I haven't been involved. Even though I know all this and have asked time and time again for a copy and to be involved in reviewing it this does not happen. My care would be far more effective if I was involved. I know what support I need and what I don't need help with. My support needs change over time and that's why the care plan is designed to be reviewed regularly. I have just come out of hospital and all my medication has changed and the support I now need is very different than from before my admission. Although I have accessed the services for 15 years now I think I have received 2 copies of my care plan in all that time."

What types of therapies are currently available within the Mental Health Services?

Mental health services are provided at both primary and secondary level.

Primary Care includes:
- GP surgery
- Local hospital
- Walk-in centre

Secondary Care run by specialist mental health staff includes:
- Care in the community
- Day hospitals and centres
- Drop-in centres
- In-patient clinics
- 24 hour helplines
- Crisis provision

Care provided at both levels can include:
- Drug treatment
- Talking therapies
- Psychotherapy
- Art therapy

Because some service users have complex conditions, care in the community will often be treated with a combination of therapies, i.e. medication and counselling. Some complementary therapies such as acupuncture are now being used alongside more traditional methods. Many people experiencing mental health difficulties find many complementary therapies very beneficial, especially as they have virtually no side-effects. There is increasing evidence about the effectiveness of these therapies in this area.

One talking therapy which is increasingly used is **Cognitive Behaviour Therapy (CBT).**

Cognitive Behaviour Therapy is a way of talking about how you think about yourself, the world and other people; how what you do affects your thoughts and feelings.

CBT can help you change how you think ('Cognitive') and what you do ('Behaviour'). These changes can help you to feel better. Unlike some of the other talking treatments, it focuses on your 'here and now' problems and difficulties. Instead of focusing on the causes of your distress or symptoms *in the past*, it looks for ways to improve your state of mind *in the present*.

It has been found to be helpful in:

- Anxiety
- Depression
- Panic
- Agoraphobia and other phobias
- Social phobia
- Bulimia
- Obsessive Compulsive Disorder
- Post Traumatic Stress Disorder
- Schizophrenia

How does CBT work?

CBT can help you make sense of overwhelming problems by breaking them down into smaller parts. This makes it easier to see how they are connected and how they affect you. These parts are:

- Situation - a problem, event or difficult circumstance
From this can follow:
- Thoughts
- Emotions
- Physical feelings
- Actions

Each of these areas can affect the others. How you think about a problem can affect how you feel, physically and emotionally. It can also alter what you do about it.

There is some debate about the effectiveness of CBT but there is increasing evidence to show that it is not the *type* of therapy that is important but rather the quality of the relationship between patient and therapist.

As mental health service users and their supporters continue to fight for a wider range of treatments, I hope that drug therapy will become the treatment at the *end* of the line instead of at the beginning.

For people with severe and enduring mental illness, the care package may need to include help with social skills, plus work to address their social isolation. It is reported that 1-in-4 service users have no contact with their families and 1-in-3 have no contact with friends.

"Service users themselves believe that adequate housing and income and assistance with the social and occupational aspects of daily living are among the most important aspects of care."
(*National Mental Health Service Framework, p 46*)

Mental health continuum

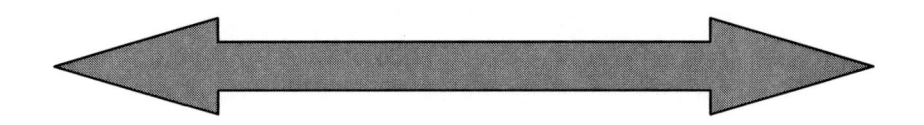

Poor Mental Health   **Good Mental health**

The mental health continuum diagram above is simply a representation of a scale on which our mental health can vary. Some days my mental health is poor and on other days it is good. Some days I will move across the line above from good to poor and in between. What I am trying to say here is that measuring mental health is not black or white, it's more grey *and* black *and* white.

Given enough stress we can all experience poor mental health. It is just that some people have had a variety of experiences and vulnerabilities that contribute to this stress. Dehydration, sleep deprivation, overworking and many other factors can trigger stress. I know in myself that if I reduce my stress levels, then I increase my mental well-being and I can cope.

I find it hard to understand why the mental health acute wards are such stressful places because surely this does not help anyone's mental well-being, be it patients' or staff's. I also can't understand why mental health services don't have more holistic and complementary therapies. I have tried acupuncture, aromatherapy and massage and all help me cope with my life.

Physical health and mental health

Physical health and mental health are intertwined. Most people know that when they are feeling physically unwell their mental health suffers as well. Feeling physically unwell can reduce your confidence, your concentration and your ability to cope.

The reverse is also true in that when you feel mentally unwell your physical health suffers. Feeling depressed can lead to not eating, not taking exercise and avoiding others. There is a lot of research about the links between physical and mental health.

There is also a lot of evidence to show that if you have a mental health diagnosis then you're more likely to have physical health needs—which may go unchecked and unmet.

People with severe mental health needs die 10 years younger than other people because of poor physical health.

The association between mental illness and poor physical health has long been recognised. The *British Medical Journal* first reported this relationship over 60 years ago. Current research confirms that to this day patients in psychiatric services have high rates of physical illness, much of which is still going undetected.

People with schizophrenia and bipolar disorders have higher risks of certain physical conditions than average:
- 2 to 4 times the rate of cardiovascular diseases
- 2 to 4 times the rate of respiratory diseases
- 5 times the rate of diabetes
- 8 times the rate of Hepatitis C

Maslow and the hierarchy of needs

The humanistic psychologist Abraham Maslow, in his 1943 paper A Theory of Human Motivation, defined a hierarchy of five levels of basic human needs. He believed that human beings strive for an upper level of capabilities and that each level of need has to be satisfied before the person is able to focus on the next level. So we all work from the bottom of the triangle upwards towards self-actualisation.

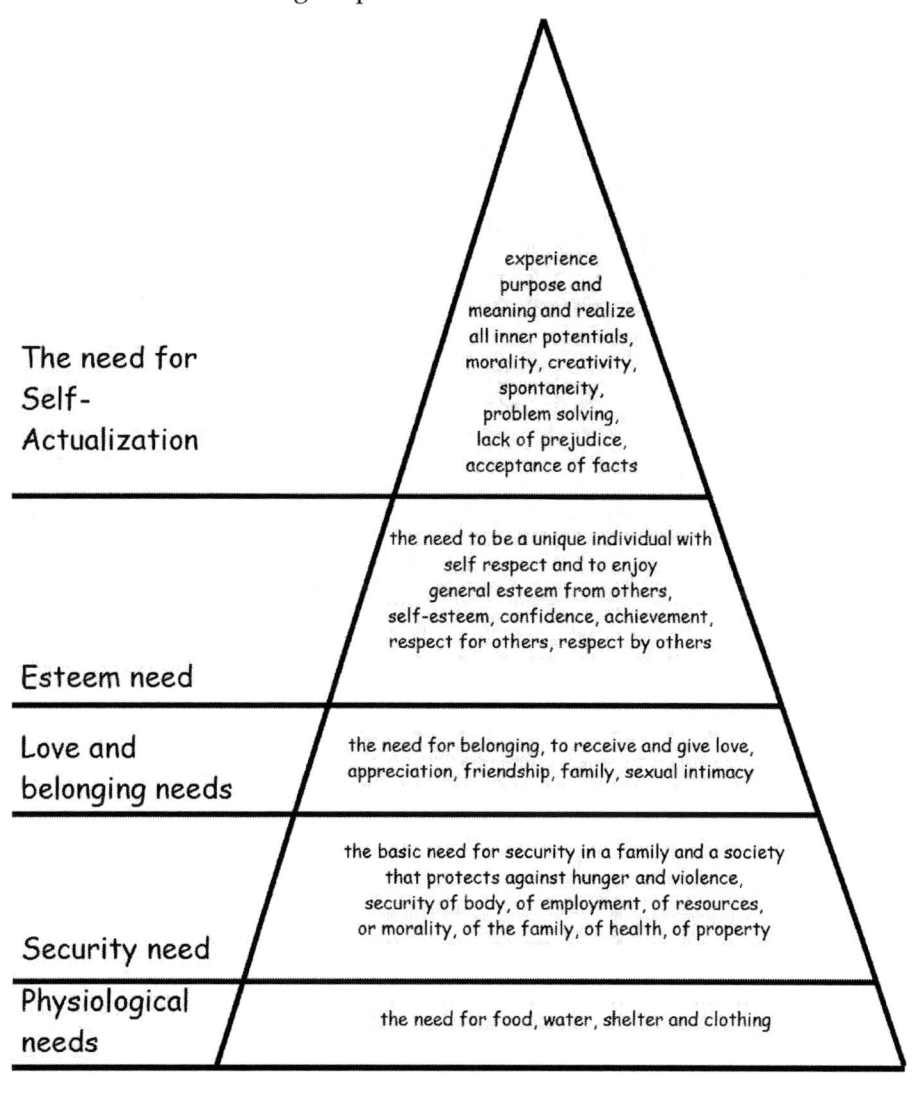

The need for Self-Actualization: experience purpose and meaning and realize all inner potentials, morality, creativity, spontaneity, problem solving, lack of prejudice, acceptance of facts

Esteem need: the need to be a unique individual with self respect and to enjoy general esteem from others, self-esteem, confidence, achievement, respect for others, respect by others

Love and belonging needs: the need for belonging, to receive and give love, appreciation, friendship, family, sexual intimacy

Security need: the basic need for security in a family and a society that protects against hunger and violence, security of body, of employment, of resources, or morality, of the family, of health, of property

Physiological needs: the need for food, water, shelter and clothing

I am currently studying psychology and I realised, looking at this diagram, why most of the current mental health services do not work properly. Mental health services work on the principle that you need to change your thoughts and behaviour and increase your coping strategies in order to deal with the distress, mostly through the use of medication. However it is really hard, if not impossible, for someone who does not have their *basic needs* satisfied to work on any of their thoughts and think about developing new ways of coping. They need to work on the bottom of the triangle before they can move up.

Where does somebody go to get help with their finances or their housing needs? What support do they need to access services out there? For an example I will look at the issues of housing and finance. I know that most people from mental health residential services end up in council flats in the inner city, and those discharged from mental health acute wards have unsuitable homes to return to. How can you maintain a state of positive mental health when you are living from day to day in fear of others in your community, or in uncertainty about whether you are going to have a roof over your head?

Finances are neglected when you feel bad and a lot of people I know are financially unstable. Where is the support? When I left university I lost my home, money and security, my independence and my future career and quite quickly lost all my friends except one. If I hadn't had my parents to fall back on I would not have had a home when I left hospital.

So again, by looking at Maslow's hierarchy of needs, I can see how the basic building blocks of life, for someone like me, consist of essential lower foundations *that are unsupported*. Aren't these the areas that people with mental health difficulties need practical support with? I know I did; I know my friends did; and I know a lot of people who can't move forward towards recovery because they do not have the practical support.

When I left hospital in 2005 I was determined to move forward, so I rented a place with support from my family and now I have a place I can feel safe in and call my home. I am slowly building up my network of friends again, but I would have liked to support with this too.

This kind of practical support either needs to be fought for from the mental health services or comes from my fellow peers (people with experience of mental health difficulties who have started self-help groups) or other voluntary organisations. *Framework* offers this support, but due to insufficient funding it is time-limited and they are overrun with people needing their help.

Active, practical support is vital in helping people move forward.

Stress and Vulnerability

Vulnerabilities Physical poor health Childhood Self-harm Bulimia Anxiety	*Personal protectors* Good coping mechanisms No drugs or alcohol Positive outlook The glass is half full Meaning and purpose in life
Environmental stressors Medication side-effects Stigma surrounding diagnosis	*Environmental protectors* Safe and secure home Family and friendships Self-help group and other peer support Flexible voluntary work Reasonable level of intelligence

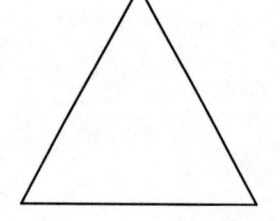

It's like a balancing act

This type of diagram is used by some mental health workers to look at vulnerabilities, stressors and protective factors (personal and environmental). If you have used SWOT diagrams (Strengths, Weaknesses, Opportunities and Threats), you will be familiar with using this type of grid for other purposes.

I have filled it out for my personal circumstances, and although I originally included far more in each box I have tried to keep it simple here. The titles for each box are a guide, but the key thing is to think broadly in each area. For example, medication/smoking/alcohol might be a stressor *and* a protective factor. Every individual will be able to fill theirs out differently and can include a wide variety of areas/factors specific to that person.

I have included this diagram as I found it a really useful tool to help me identify the areas that have helped me in my life and the areas that have caused me difficulties. Although I recognize there are some areas I have identified in this chart where there is nothing I can change, such as childhood experiences, there are many things on here I could change.

The contents of the two boxes on the left worsened my mental health and the two on the right helped me cope. If I could decrease the stressors and limit the effects of my vulnerabilities, and at the same time increase and maintain the protective factors, I would be more likely to remain well.

Completing this diagram helped me to become aware of all the factors affecting my mental health. It was refreshing to do as previously all emphasis by mental health services had been on my weaknesses and the need for medication as the only source of support. It has helped me to see that I have a lot of strengths and coping strategies already, and by identifying vulnerabilities and stressors I could work on these areas. It gave me a fuller picture of what helped and hindered my wellbeing. I could also use this diagram to talk with the people supporting me about what help I needed, and why, and in turn it helped them to understand the whole picture and what was important for me.

My first encounter with the Mental Health System

Where do you start?

The first port of call, people would assume, should be your GP, but I didn't think of that at the time because the difficulties I was going through were emotional difficulties and I thought my GP was there just for physical problems.

When I went to my GP I had no confidence that s/he would understand. If you have kept your problems to yourself, not confided in anyone, even your own family, it's hard to think that someone unknown to you can even begin to understand.

It's also a problem that doctors just don't have the time to sit there and *listen*. Most GPs—not all, there are some brilliant GPs out there—don't understand mental health or mental health difficulties or a cry for help when they hear one.

When I first knew I needed help I just wanted someone to talk things through with, about the abuse and my childhood. I went to my GP but didn't know what to say, so I waffled about other things and never really said what I needed to.

The importance of admitting you have a problem

Admitting that something is wrong is the first and vital step, but I hadn't really done that. I knew something wasn't right; the drinking had got out of control and my self-harming was more extreme, but I didn't know where to turn. I just wanted someone to talk things through with and that happened to be my GP's nurse. It was she who took that extra time to enquire how I was. She was gentle and kind whenever she saw me and took things slowly. She didn't force me to see the GP but asked if I wanted her to talk to him first, and also suggested which GP I should see. Some GPs, as you might already know, are better at some aspects of their job than others. Some GPs like the elderly, some the young and some mental health and wellbeing.

The first step for me was having someone who cared and wanted to help and took the time to listen to what I wanted and needed, and it was the nurse who supplied that initially. There was no pressure and no judgement on the nurse's part; she just wanted to help.

When I first received help

My first visit was actually to a psychologist following my rape at 15. When I first tried to get help I didn't know where to go or who to turn to. I actually spoke to a teacher at my secondary school and she didn't know.

Although the school made sure I saw someone, it was wary of attracting attention to the fact I needed help. Any such incident might reflect badly on the school if it became known. So I had to cross town to go and see a psychologist. Because I felt forced to see her, the therapeutic relationship was never good and I stopped going as soon as I could.

Referral to a Psychiatrist

James Thurber, 1962: "I do not have a psychiatrist and I do not want one for the simple reason that if he listened to me long enough he might end up disturbed."

My first visit

This was about three years after last accessing any support from the psychologist and was during my last year at university. Seeing him for the first time was scary and unnerving. I paced the entrance hall. I didn't want to go in. My head was full of questions, buzzing with thoughts and concerns. What would he think of me? Would he lock me up? Should I even be here? I wanted to get out of that place as soon as I entered. Those five minutes' waiting seemed at the time the longest of my life.

I was called through and he seemed nice, but where was the couch I had expected? Don't all psychiatrists have couches? Instead there were three chairs and I was shown to one. Forty minutes went fast. I felt guarded, as if my every word was being examined—which it was, of course. I came out with a prescription for antidepressants I did not want but felt obliged to take, as if some magic tablet might help take away the distress. Forty minutes had passed so quickly and resulted in what? A box of pills.

The problem with being diagnosed

When I entered the system again after my breakdown at university, I didn't receive any diagnosis for a long time. At first it was 'clinical depression with panic disorder' and then over the years it changed from diagnosis to diagnosis, all varying in degree, some seemingly worse than others.

Not knowing what was wrong was the hardest bit, the never-ending waiting to be told 'you're MAD'!! In the beginning I didn't think I was ill—I was just struggling with life. Soon that conviction was washed away by the tablets and the side-effects and the stigma. Receiving a diagnosis meant receiving a label that shouted to everyone that I couldn't cope. It didn't help that the label kept changing, and with the changing diagnosis society's changing view of me, all of which made it a hundred times worse. I already felt different. Being told I was different because of mental health difficulties just compounded that feeling.

I had gone from having my own home, a life, some friends and a future, to having less than nothing. The few friends I had could not cope with my changing moods, my bizarre behaviours and thoughts, and slowly, one by one they disappeared. I had to leave my flat and move back to my parents and was eventually admitted to hospital. My future career as a teacher was gone.

If all this happened to you in the space of weeks, even without mental health difficulties, how well would you cope?

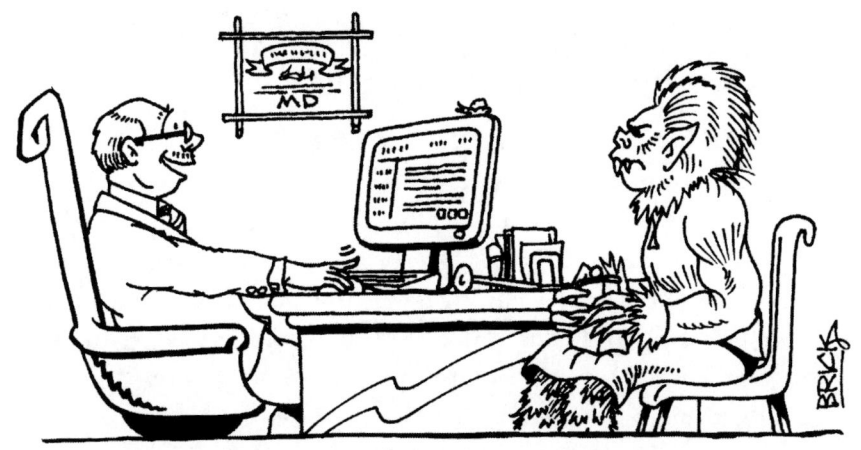

"And how are you getting on with the new pills?"

Medication

Urghhh. I hate my medication. Don't get me wrong, it can help some people and helps take the edge off my distress at times, but the other effects that it has are *not* good.

What effects have drugs had on me?

Over the last fifteen years I've taken a wide variety of prescribed medication. Each time you go on a drug you have to give your body time to adjust. Every time you're taken off an individual drug it has an effect on you. Every time your medication is switched it has an effect on you, your mind and your body.

I have taken antidepressants, antipsychotics, sedatives, sleeping-tablets and a range of medication for my physical health. I am addicted emotionally and physically to the sedatives and sleeping tablets. I have been on the highest possible dose of antidepressants and although as an in-patient they should be closely monitored, they weren't.

Possible dangerous reactions to drugs

The side-effects of the higher doses of antipsychotics have been distressing in themselves. They have numbed me down so much I can't think at all, even to make a cup of tea. The agitation and the need to constantly move attract the stares of other people and the aching intensity in the joints that I get, even on the lower doses, is horrible. Then there is the constant salivation and the soaking wet pillow every morning and the vivid nightmares and dreams. I have had other physical effects as well such as high blood-pressure, and I experienced a reaction to one drug I was given that was actually life-threatening. My muscles contracted into spasms, which required emergency admission and treatment.

Then there are the mood changes that became so apparent on one particular drug that I had to come off it, taking months for me to return to my usual self. If I come off any of the drugs I have to cope with horrendous withdrawal effects which again take months if not years to get over. One drug I still have to take today because I can't seem to withdraw from it at all without becoming acutely ill in the withdrawal process, no matter how slowly I do it.

For me the effects of the medications that are positive are very limited and are mostly concerned with helping me get enough sleep. When I have needed to take an overdose they of course then come in handy! But the distressing effects far outweigh the positive.

The side-effects to medication are one of the reasons that people with mental health problems find it difficult, if not impossible, to commit to regular, full-time or even part-time work.

Admission to an in-patient facility

Between 1989 and 1990, 16,300 people were given compulsory treatment against their will.
"In 2000-2001, 26,707 were formally admitted against their will, in addition to 19,750 who went voluntarily into hospital in the first instance but *who were then sectioned*.
In 2006-07 there were 20,400 detentions after informal admission to hospital. This compares with 20,000 in 2005-06"(NHS Statistics).

What's the difference between voluntary admission and being sectioned?

My first admission into hospital was as a voluntary patient. Basically I either went in voluntarily or I would have been sectioned and forced onto the ward.

Where was the voluntary bit, you ask? I still question that.

If you were going away for a weekend course where you didn't know the location or the people and you'd lost the joining instructions, then you just might be anxious about what would happen! Imagine how that would be, magnified for me by the element of coercion and powerlessness, no experience of what was likely to happen and being already in a very distressed state.

What do I take?

Will everyone be like me?

What will the patients and staff be like?

Will I be safe?

Will I share a room?

What will the therapy be?

First impressions of the unit

The corridor I walked down seemed like a dark tunnel to the unknown. I had my parents on either side guiding me as I walked. Places had become unreal and finding my direction was hard. I felt consumed by emotion and didn't want to be there. I wanted to die, but I wasn't here for me. I was here for my family because of their concern.

Dying for me at this point would have been a relief and an escape from the depths of despair. Depression is not the Monday blues or that feeling of being a bit down. No, this was THERE IS NO WAY OUT. That tunnel with the light at the end that people talk about? This had no light and it felt, instead of there being light, that I had fallen into a deep pit that caved in every time I tried to climb out until I no longer tried.

This place at the end of the corridor was the only hope for my parents to feel they had done their best and that I would be safe. They had found me self-harming again, something they still do not understand. I needed the self-harm to relieve the distress—but to continue to survive, *not* to die. The voices I heard that others could not were my sanctuary, although at times they could also be distressing, and confused even further my thoughts and anxieties.

The panic ran through my body when I saw the door. I didn't want to go in. The staff were expecting me, though, and ushered me into the entrance room where I sat and waited. The panic would not go away and I started to hyperventilate, breathing quicker and quicker. My heart pounding through my chest felt as if it was about to burst. I have had panic attacks many times before and even though I knew I wasn't going to die and that it would eventually fade away, it felt like this every time it happened.

I was taken into a small room and interviewed for what seemed hours, but apparently it was only 20 minutes. I was asked about my self-harm and the voices and any other difficulties I was experiencing, but I was not in a fit state physically or emotionally to express myself clearly.

Life on the unit

It took me days to work out where everything was, including the toilet and where to go to get a drink of tea. When I could eventually talk to them I relied heavily on other patients for information. I was told little by the nurses and weeks passed before I even knew I could be escorted by my parents off the ward for a walk. Going for a walk was an invaluable respite from the ward, even though the car parks I walked became dull and tiresome.

The view from the window of the room I was in was of those same car parks and I began to pass the time observing the regular visitors and staff. I watched their cars leave, wishing I could go with them. I was so bored at times and so tired at others. The main focus of the day was mealtimes with little else to do in between.

On one of my stays on the ward both my Gran and my dog died. I heard the staff discussing that they wouldn't tell me in case I couldn't deal with it. Since they were my two best friends then of course it would upset me. But were they and my parents right to lie to me about the events?

It turned out that both Gran and my dog were fine. It was all an hallucination. Even so, the staff never came up to me to ask if I was okay. They just observed from around corners. I was too scared to ask to talk to them yet they still insisted *I* must approach *them* to tell them everything. They were strangers to me and I knew that everything I said would be written down and discussed at meetings. My life was open to anyone who wanted to delve in. I am a very private person and I don't want my life open to all.

They wanted me to go to occupational therapy and make another plate. It must have been the fiftieth. I used to like pottery but now I hate it. Time goes so slowly when you're on the ward.

Imagine being in a room you are not familiar with, with nothing to do. Everything has been removed that might be 'dangerous' for you, or distracting. No television or radio, no computer, nothing to read, not able to make your own drinks or food. In fact, imagine not being allowed to do anything without someone to watch what you do 24/7, and knowing that they're taking notes about your behaviour whether you scratch your nose, walk up and down, sigh or anything else you do when you're bored.

Every few hours they'd bring you a tablet to take that 'will make you feel better'. And you have no choice about taking it.

That's life on an acute ward.

What I hoped for on the unit

What I longed for was the therapy I needed, that person to talk to, none of which existed. The only thing I did get was constant observation and drugs, endless drugs. These drugs were even more intense than before and made me feel worse than I had when I was first admitted. The nurses said the effects would wear off and that I would get used to them, but I didn't. My legs felt so weighted down they would not go in the direction I wanted.

The agitation intensified and I needed to keep moving, even if it meant I walked up and down the small ward most of the day. My vision blurred and I felt intolerably nauseous for most of the time. When I did sit I clock-watched the minutes and seconds that passed so slowly, and even time itself seemed to slow down with the passing of days and weeks.

What benefit did I get from being on the ward?

I left that ward still with my anxiety, depression and hallucinations but so drugged to the eyeballs that I could not think about them and did not care. I had been medicated so much I had become a different person—a quiet, subdued and easily manipulated person.

Was it the effect of the drugs or the effect of being locked away for so long from everything that was familiar and real?

After I left the unit

I no longer knew what I wanted or needed from life. Everything was all one, long, big blur and all I wanted to do was sleep in my own bed, stroke my own dog and be somewhere I felt safe.

Had I left with post-traumatic stress disorder? Probably. Had the treatment helped me reach the causes of my distress and help me overcome them? No! It had ignored the problem, drugged the symptoms and caused me to fear ever going on the ward again, so ultimately causing more problems than it solved.

However, I continued to tell myself that the doctors were always right, that they knew what they were doing, that I had to get worse before I got better, as the psychiatrists explained. At that time I foolishly believed them. I am stronger now and I am more confident and able to stand up for what I believe, but it has taken me ten years to become *me* again. It took me six of those years to fight to see a psychologist rather than a psychiatrist and at the same time receive help for physical health needs that had been ignored (and which I only managed by going to a private hospital).

Right from the beginning I was the one who *knew what I needed*; someone to talk to, to believe in me and support me through the past distress. If only I had been listened to back then instead of being subdued by their chemical cosh!

Conclusions

I suppose the reason the mental health system is so based on the medical model, so biased towards the physical, is because they think that all the causes of mental health problems must have a pathological basis, a chemical imbalance in the brain rather than being some distress you've experienced that continues to affect you.

Yes, there might be some underlying biological factors—some biological predisposition that makes you more vulnerable, or susceptible towards mental health problems. But all the people I know who have mental health difficulties suffer because of distressing experiences in their past or some unresolved issues that they need to work through. I'm not completely anti-medication, but neither am I all for it. Medication should be the *last* resort not the first.

What support have I received from the mental health services and what was it like?

Some services I have received from the mental health system have been good. When I finally started seeing a psychologist in 2004 and was allocated a supportive community psychiatric nurse, things started to change. For the first time in my life I felt I was being heard. I could talk openly to the psychologist about the distress and the voices and from then on I started to move forward. It was the help I had always needed.

The community nurse listened to me as an equal human being, gave me back control over my life, believed I could achieve what I wanted to achieve in life and saw my potential. He saw a future for me and had hope. Along the way I have met other like-minded individuals who have also seen me as a person in my own right, but they have been few and far between. I must mention however, one nurse who was an inspiration to me. It was that nurse who described me as 'wonderfully strange'. But it wasn't this statement that changed my life; it was something else he said.

The nurse asked me, "What do you want out of life? What are your dreams?"

At first I said I had none and that they had been taken away from me, but then I began to think more and more about what I had wanted.

He then said, "Why not follow those dreams?" WHY NOT? I came up with lots of excuses such as I could no longer work with children because of the label I had been given, but the phrase WHY NOT? kept coming back to me.

Why couldn't I do the things I wanted to do? Why couldn't I have dreams? And why couldn't I follow them? Just like anybody else I *needed* to have dreams to follow, a purpose and a reason to live again.

From that day on, I did!! I followed my dreams and it's changed my life completely!

Direct payments for care

Stephen Ladyman, MP, 2003: "If we make people's personal ambitions, people's own desires and hopes and dreams the centre of planning the support they need, we liberate people, we transform lives, we make things possible that previously seemed impossible. Let's make sure that we get that message out there to every single person who is using care services in this country."

The purpose of direct payments is to give recipients control over their own lives by providing an alternative to the social care services provided by local councils. The financial payment gives the person flexibility to look beyond off-the-peg services.

Now the system is organised in the same way that care for the elderly is managed. The person can have their own funding account and buy in the services they think they need.

Diary: 11 February 2004
"I am hopefully going to get direct payments to buy in my own services. I'd like to buy into the Voluntary Car Scheme with a worker to help get me places and help me be more confident travelling. Then I won't be so reliant on my parents for transport. I just about get to the post office and round the short block, on good days.

It is still anxiety provoking. My legs have been hurting as well. It all seems a tremendous effort and every day I have the struggle just to get up and face the day."

It is now 2008, four years since I have been trying to achieve a direct payment assessment, which is just the first stage before applying. I have been unable to get an NHS assessment as nobody seems to have the right training and there is anyway not enough in the Social Services' budget, even if I prove to be eligible. Funding would have to be taken from other services to afford the direct payments.

Diary: December 2008
"I am hoping to become one of two trial subjects for the instruction of personal individual budgets (similar to direct payments). Apparently every person accessing social care through Social Services will be offered an individual budget. My concern is that this will create a two-tier service with some receiving a high level of support and others a very poor service. Funding will be taken away from statutory services such as day centres so as to fund these budgets. This is a good idea in principle but is probably not workable in practice; but I will keep an open mind."

I think that direct payments/individual budgets will work well for people with mental health difficulties under the following conditions:

1. If they could use the system without a struggle
2. If they could find properly-trained personal assistants once they have received the payments
3. If they have the appropriate support and advice to be able to carry out both the above

This hasn't been helped by the fact that the local support service designed to help people access direct payments has been replaced by a national support service. (This was probably due to the fact that the original service actually helped people to access direct payments and highlighted the need for easier access to and information about direct payments for those with mental health difficulties, and also helped them cut costs and services at the same time.)

What in the mental health system hasn't helped me?

Most of my experiences of the mental health services have been poor. The services took away the control I had over my life and controlled it for me. The treatment I received in hospital was not caring and supportive but was all about risk management and control and medication enforcement.

The psychiatrists similarly only saw my case from their point of view and they needed to be in control. Most of the time I was not listened to about what I needed, or wanted. Conversations were one way and involvement in my own care was at best token, and at worst non-existent. I was labelled and put in a box and if I argued with them or tried to debate with them about my care I was labelled as attention-seeking or as having a personality disorder. If my parents challenged them they were seen as controlling and manipulative. I was the lowest of the low and did not matter. When your self-esteem is already at rock bottom this way of being dealt with can't possibly help you.

What happened to me on the acute unit and afterwards still affects my emotions and depresses me. I would not and do not like to think that other people will continue to go through the same experiences I had on those acute wards.

It has taken me a long time to come to terms with all the events, some of which you would not believe, that happened on that ward, both to me and to other people. I still vividly remember being pinned down and injected for daring to argue with a nurse over my treatment.

I remember the lack of respect that most of the nurses had for me and the times I needed and asked to talk to a nurse, yet they would tell me 'just another half an hour' or 'wait till tomorrow'.

Current Crisis Provision

In 1999 the National Service Framework prescribed the need for 24 hour crisis provision. Before the implementation of the Crisis Resolution and Home Treatment teams there was no mental health service provision outside of the usual working hours. If you needed help out of hours there was no one to call upon except for the normal Accident and Emergency services and Social Services' out of hour's service. There was also no opportunity when experiencing a crisis to have treatment at home, so hospital admission was the only option if you were at serious risk to yourself or others. Many voluntary organisations plugged the gap by setting up out of hours helplines but these were usually limited. The government set out to form 335 Crisis Resolution and Home Treatment teams by December 2004. It was hoped that bed usage would be reduced and that with mental health workers working with people at home, they could tackle the cause of the crisis, thus reducing the recovery time needed and minimising further crises while maintaining the individual's independence and control over their own care.

Crisis Resolution and Home Treatment teams are broken down into two types of support. The crisis resolution part is a community-based team providing rapid access for assessment of someone thought to be experiencing a mental health crisis. The home treatment part of the service provides time-limited, intensive home support.

There have been mixed reports about the effectiveness of these new teams. Currently the majority of research has been based purely on number crunching e.g. bed usage. This type of research does not give a full picture of what is happening within services. There have been many people who have had poor experiences of the Crisis Resolution and Home Treatment teams, but it was important to find out if this was just the minority of cases or was more widespread, and if the latter, to find out what areas needed to be improved. It was important also to find out what it was that helped people who were experiencing a crisis.

I therefore decided to find out by conducting some research into the patient's experience of having a mental health crisis and of using the Crisis Resolution and Home Treatment teams. Along with a mixed team of people who use services, carers, academics and research staff, we conducted 36 interviews with people who had recently used one of these teams. What we found really does make common sense.

Common sense about what helps and hinders recovery: a brief summary

What we found helped recovery, whether this was from staff or from friends and family or other sources of support, was how important it was to experience the following:

- *Reassurance*

Just knowing someone was there, either in person or contactable at the end of the phone, who had some understanding of what was happening

- *Positive relationships that showed*

consistency, acceptance, understanding, listening and hearing, and that were non-judgemental

- *The service user enabled and involved in recovery*

Having control over their own life and making their own decisions and choice over their treatment all helped recovery.

- *Other factors:*

General practitioners

Having a supportive, non-judgemental GP proved to be helpful

- *Practical support*

Having practical help with household tasks, shopping, cleaning, gardening and also help with childcare, helped remove excess pressure

- *Access and flexibility*

Having access to support, whether it was services, family or friends, that was flexible so that it met their needs at the time it was needed

What we found hindered recovery was:

- *Negative attitudes and behaviour*

Again this was from anyone, staff or services, friends, family or the community

- *Expectations prior to crisis support*

This was the individual's expectations of the service that they expected to receive. Both low and high expectations affected their perceptions of the quality of the service and support that they received.

- *Lack of continuity*

This was lack of continuity from staff, friends, family, GPs or other sources of support e.g. church. Having regular contact and visits with someone was important.

- *Lack of appropriate/organised follow-up*

This point related only to the services. There were long waiting times for referrals to other services e.g. psychology and other therapies, and in addition there was a lack of follow-up after being discharged or even when still accessing the services. There were also gaps in service provision i.e. between someone being discharged from the Crisis Resolution and Home Treatment teams and when they could access other services for longer-term support.

All in all what the results really show is that it is not rocket science to help someone who is experiencing a mental health crisis. Having someone who develops a good relationship with you; accepts you; listens; is non-judgemental; is consistent; involves you all the way; provides reassurance and helps practically; these are the main things that help someone during a crisis. Where family and friends didn't have much knowledge of mental health it didn't matter provided they were prepared to listen and hear what the person him/herself was going through, learning and adapting along the way.

The acute ward again

I had hoped things would have changed for the better, but only this year I was admitted to the psychiatric acute ward and found to my horror that things had got worse. I could not believe that the wards could get worse but they had. Yes, they had had a lick of paint, some new furniture and a restyling but they were the worst place to be when feeling mentally fragile. Even my friends and relatives could not bear to stay for long.

Staff morale is so low now that they don't challenge their managers and they seem to have accepted that nothing will change. The smoking ban means that staffing is cut by half on the ward as many staff members are needed to escort patients from the ward to have a smoke outside. Staff inevitably end up using this power of being able to take patients for a smoke or not as a reward or punishment and as a means of control.

Food on the ward has never been good but some of the food this time was inedible. I am vegetarian and have been most of my life and twice during one week went without a meal due to the lack of a vegetarian option. I know that it can be hard to cater for all needs but the catering service can provide most options if the staff ask. The staff knew I was vegetarian and when there was not a vegetarian option for a third time in that same week, I insisted that they ring and request one (I was lucky that I was feeling a little stronger and that there was an amenable nurse on duty at the time.)

The ward this time was filthy. Yes, they had cleaners but they weren't really bothered and didn't really clean. Patches of dirt on the floor remained there all week and the cleaners used only a slightly damp mop to lightly sweep the floor. Apparently they were not allowed to move the furniture, so some areas never got cleaned. The edges between the floor and the wall were black and the grime on the doors was sticky black. In fact one patient became so fed up with putting his hand on the mucky door that he cleaned it himself. People aren't well on the ward and will cause spillages of all varieties but these should always be cleaned up as soon as they are spotted or reported. Blood remained on the floor for over a day and a large patch of urine in the phone box which, even though I had let the staff know was there, meant I had to let them know again two hours later as it still hadn't been cleaned up.

There were two small kitchen areas for making drinks. The mugs we used were plastic and were ingrained a dirty brown. These areas were piled with dirty mugs, plates and bowls and the surface was covered in sugar and milk. I tried to clean the kitchen area but was told off by a member of staff as apparently 'it will only get dirty again'. I asked if she discouraged every patient from cleaning up after themselves and she said yes. I said that if she discouraged every patient not to clean then yes, it would become this bad again. Sitting next to it was making me ill and tidying up gave me something productive to do.

There is nothing to do on the ward besides sit, sleep, read or make cups of tea, watching the clock and waiting for the next meal or psychiatric review. Occupational therapy used to happen on the ward two, sometimes even three, times a day, which was not enough then, and now even the occupational therapist is constrained by what s/he can do and usually there is only one activity a day, if that. Understaffed and underfunded, how can they do their job? Many of the occupational therapists become frustrated and feel undervalued and soon leave.

The culture on the ward is very different from the world outside. There is a ranking of power from manager and psychiatrist at the top down to the nursing staff, then to the other staff and finally with no power at all the patients and carers. As a patient this is frustrating and you learn or are told by other patients how to get what you need. Playing by their rules is the key. Doing what they say is the quickest way to get out, even if it makes you worse and you have to deal with the problems incurred when you're finally out. Don't show any extremes of emotion, anger or upset, even if they a realistic. If you're not allowed to have your cigarettes to go for a smoke, or pain relief medication to ease a physical pain, even when they know about the physical difficulties you have, you have to hold your frustration back and ask again and again but calmly.

I have been in pain with my gall bladder for just under a year and as anybody who has gallstones will know, they are excruciating. I was being prescribed painkillers, Ibuprofen, by my general practitioner for months before I went into hospital. However, as soon as you are admitted with mental health problems the pain is not seen by the staff as real, even when you have an ultra-sound scan to prove the problem exists. I was now questioned every time I needed them. Why did I need them? Where was the pain? And I had to explain again and again. It was a battle each time to get the pain relief I needed. When I finally got the Ibuprofen, on most occasions I then had to try and get some food to take it with. I lost count of the number of times I was asked by nurses 'why do you need something to eat with Ibuprofen?' As it states on every box, Ibuprofen should be taken with or after food as it can cause stomach cramps and ulcers. I explained this each time and once was told by a nurse 'Well, I have taken it without food and I haven't had a problem.' Taking it as a one-off probably wouldn't be too bad but I have to take it regularly. This 'advice' is anyway not something a qualified nurse should be giving.

Not knowing what support was available to me or what was written on my care plan is another area that has hindered my recovery. Even though I have asked for a copy of my current plan, I have still not received one.

Guidance for Users

Standard 4 *(National Mental Health Service Framework, p 41)*
All mental health service users on a CPA (Care Programme Approach) should:

- Receive care which optimises engagement, anticipates or prevents a crisis, and reduces risk
- Have a copy of a written care plan which:
    - includes the action to be taken in a crisis by the service user, their carer, and their care co-ordinator
    - advises their GP how they should respond if the service user needs additional help
    - is regularly reviewed by their care co-ordinator
    - provides for access to services 24 hours a day, 365 days a year

Day to day living

If I had known early on that I could get psychotherapy, would I still have gone through these later years of crisis? Would the distress have been so ingrained?

If I had been given a copy of my care plan and, even better, been involved in it from the start, I could have had a say in how I would like to be treated and my treatment would have been so much more effective. At this point I must say that I now have a great community nurse who involves me in all decision-making and who *follows* what I need rather than *telling* me what I need. I hope that more staff will follow this approach, but I know from other people who use the services that this is generally not yet the case.

Practical support can at times be even more important than emotional support and talking. When I was moving into my new place and living on my own for the first time, talking about how I would cope was important but not as important as helping with the stress of the actual move. I had no furniture, no money and none of the essentials. I had never had a home of my own. I didn't know how to pay bills or how to read the meter—all simple things other people take for granted. I needed someone to help me with all these things. I couldn't even catch a bus or go to the local shop on my own because I suffered from panic attacks.

I needed to work on all these everyday jobs, and no matter how much talking and listening and advising is done, *practical* support is essential in overcoming these hurdles if the move is to be a success. Fortunately I had support from a voluntary organisation and my family and friends.

Difference between a psychologist and a psychiatrist

A friend of mine said to me that a psychiatrist was trained to see a condition and a diagnosis and a psychologist was trained to look at the whole person, and that's very true.

A psychiatrist is first trained as a doctor and then receives training in mental health. They look at your case-notes, conduct a brief assessment on your presenting symptoms and then make a diagnosis which informs the treatment given (usually medication). Only a psychiatrist or doctor is qualified to prescribe drugs.

Getting to see a psychologist even now is very difficult. I waited 6 years for an appointment. When I met my second psychologist it was fantastic because he said to me that while he might have lots of fancy degrees and letters behind his name, that didn't mean a thing. I was quite shocked because I thought that I was going there to find the answers so I could get better and recover.

He said he didn't have the answers but that he wanted to work together to find the answers *with me*.

That was so different, because we were starting off on an equal footing. In fact he said that *I* was the expert on me, which had to be the right way round because it was only the third time I'd met him.

It was such a shock to find someone who was prepared to work that way and also to let me see he was human and fallible. He didn't just see the distressing symptoms that I displayed but looked for the causes behind them.

And that's what helped me move on.

Now it might be that other service users might not like that approach. They might want to be told what to do. Maybe they don't want to take responsibility for their own lives. But that is not me!

Difference between nurses, occupational therapists and social workers

Occupational therapy looks at how you occupy your days and weeks, not just as in a job but as in meaningful activity. Learning new skills or social activities could well be very beneficial to you. I had an occupational therapist in the community who was brilliant. With graded support she helped me to manage travelling on buses. For ten years I'd been unable to catch buses. You can't imagine how that limits your life. Some of the time I had hardly been able to put the bin out, let alone travel into town.

It took a lot of baby steps. First of all I would go to the door, open it and stay there until the anxiety wore off. Then I would take the bin out; then I would walk down the street; then I would go to the post office. Eventually I caught a bus with someone. Then I caught it on my own but with someone waiting at the other end; and so on and so forth.

You may be shocked to discover that this took between three and four years. I'm more independent now but it took a lot of support and time and energy from others to achieve it, as well as drawing on my own emotional energy and effort.

Unfortunately there is no steady, consistent progress in anything new I do. Even now I sometimes can't face going out. My life does not improve in one, straight, upward line. It has helped me to recognise that I am all the time improving in a general upward direction even though it is slow, and even though there are ups and downs along the way. There used to be times when I have felt deflated because I had progressed so far and then I had relapsed. What I failed to realise was that I *was* still progressing and that it was a blip and that I could learn from those blips to help me move forward. In life we all learn more from our mistakes than from our successes. The same is true when I have a blip or relapse; I can learn from this and it often propels me forward, especially when I have been stuck and unable to move on.

It takes time and patience and that is where a lot of people, family and friends and carers, run out of energy and steam to help those they love. My family and friends are vital to my wellbeing. I need them and love them but recognise the toll it takes on them emotionally and physically. There is no real support for them and it is so much needed. Voluntary carers' support groups are the only real source of support and even these are now in jeopardy with recent funding cuts. Services don't recognise the valuable support that friends, family and carers give *so freely*. Things are slowly starting to change, or is this me just hoping that they are?

Social workers

A social worker works with people who have been socially excluded or who are experiencing crisis. Their role is to provide support to enable service users to help themselves, but most of the time they are concerned with risk—the risk you pose to yourself, and to others, especially children. That tends to put a lot of service users off because they see them as hostile and not on their side.

Like nurses they have general training and then specialise in a particular area. That can produce problems. For example, someone from a Visual Impairment team came to help me regarding my eyesight. But she didn't understand that on the day she came I didn't feel well enough to do the things she asked me to do. I knew she was trying to help but she thought I was being awkward and uncooperative because I couldn't respond.

Mental health service educators

National Mental Health Service Framework, p 109: **"All education and training should be evidence-based and should stress the value of team, interdisciplinary and inter-agency working. Service users and carers should be involved in planning, providing and evaluating education and training."**

Involvement of service users in designing how the mental health system should work

There has been a drive in recent years to involve the people who use the mental health services in decision-making and in delivering care.

Areas of service-user involvement in all aspects of my local NHS Trust are increasing, including in-training, delivery, research, trust policy and care delivery itself. I myself am involved in some of this, and although I have to do it voluntarily because of being on benefits, I have personally benefited by the increase in my self-esteem and feelings of self-worth. It has given meaning to my life, and now I fight to make a difference to others.

Diary: Monday 2nd August 2004

"I managed the presentation and it was good. I was worried about the feedback but I received a letter today telling me how good it was. I am also doing a presentation at the School of Nursing. I am glad because something I really want to do is make a difference. The best way I can make a difference is by teaching others how to view mental health in a new light and find approaches that can help rather than hinder.

If I can alter just a few people's attitudes then hopefully they will change their way of working, which will have a direct and beneficial effect on the patients they treat.

This is a new opportunity and I'm excited about it. If I can draw on my experience of using services and show the impact it has had on me, then at least the pain and suffering I have been through will not have been in vain. I wish I had never received the treatment I have had from the services and from the public, but if I can use it to help things change for the better, not just for me but for others who follow, it will have been worthwhile.

I also had news today that I might be able to do one of the NHS training courses and I would be the first service user to do this. I don't think I want to work in mental health as I would find it too distressing, but I could use the training in training others."

Service users as reviewers of the service

For a few weeks I worked for the Healthcare Commission as part of a review panel that went into different NHS Trusts to review their mental health services. The commission has now become the Commission for Social Care Inspectorate and I still carry out one-day reviews for them.

I think it is essential that service users are involved in such work, but it can be very draining. When I carried out this reviewing it had to be spread out so I didn't overwhelm myself and become ill. There are many roles service users could play which would give them status and paid work but the benefits system doesn't allow for such flexibility. It's either work paid sufficiently to lift you completely out of the benefits system, or do voluntary work. For many people it's too much of a risk to commit to full-time or even part-time paid work. During my work for the Healthcare Commission I had an advisor who helped with the financial minefield, which was essential.

I prefer only to do voluntary work now because every time I have done regular paid work it has made me ill because of the expectations and the inflexibility and my lack of energy and the extreme fluctuations inherent in my condition. Becoming ill means I have to access benefits again which is always difficult, stressful and time-consuming at a very vulnerable time, contributing to a severe deterioration in my wellbeing.

Mental health service workers

It has to be acknowledged that for many years the mental health service has been the poor relation within the National Health Service. Sufficient numbers of staff are difficult to recruit and are often poorly paid, which results in high turnover rates, particularly in inner cities.

The new approaches to treatment with their multiple combinations, are not welcomed by all staff, and delivering the combination therapies demands high levels of skill and competency.

Both staff and service users are at risk of abuse, though the balance of power will always remain with the system. It's crucial that service users are involved in designing and delivering training for staff and that avenues of communication are kept open at all times.

Many workers within the system suffer from their own mental health problems. Owning up to these is dangerous, however, if they wish to progress through the system's career structure. *What does that say about the system?* It's not good, is it!

From a service user's perspective, of course, others' mental health difficulties are extra valuable because that person can relate so much better to the experience of service users. But if you have a mental health service where workers can't talk about their own mental health issues and don't feel the system helps them provide the best care, it will inevitably impact on the service users.

The Pine Project

The Pine Project, run in Nottingham, was a combination of teaching and research to evaluate the involvement of service users in the training of service staff. It's an example of the progress we can make when all the people involved in the mental health sector unite. Each party has a role to play and a voice. Service users feel that their voice has been ignored for far too long and are demanding that they play a full part in training the next generation of mental health administrators and nurses.

Because of the PINE project, service users now teach four different sessions to nurses in training:

Professionals on tap not on top: professionals can help, or they can make things more difficult. How can professionals be encouraged to help people by providing them with information and support, instead of trying to control them?

- *Diagnosis*: see the person, not the label. Everyone is an individual and everybody's mental health goes up and down, whatever diagnosis we might or might not have.

- *Living on an acute ward*: going into hospital; coming out and everything in between—experiences, survival tips and how nurses can help—taught by people who've been there.
- *Strategies for survival*: what people can do to keep well at home; what helps to cope with stress; help with spotting early signs of being unwell, or getting through a crisis.

There are encouraging responses from the trainee nurses, but we know that it will be a slow process for the *organisation* to improve as a whole.

Services need to have a radical rethink about the services they provide.

Services need to be proactive not just reactive

Services should be needs led, not service led and need to be provided locally

Support is patchy throughout the UK. Some areas have respite services (a lot are provided by voluntary services/charities) but many still do not have any. In Nottinghamshire there are no residential services at all and you have to move into the city to access a limited number of these.

There are no eating disorder services (throughout the whole of Nottingham and Nottinghamshire) besides a monthly drop-in at NHS Direct and an inpatient service for those acutely unwell and critical. Day services are limited and are being centralised. Local day services are being cut and funding limited. When funding is provided the managers have to adhere to funding rules e.g. providing work-based training and other specific groups. This means that day services can no longer provide a service at a local level, meeting the needs identified by those using the service. Instead they are told what to provide and numbers of people using the service fall because they do not help the people who access them. To work, services need to be provided locally and must be needs led. However, they are not.

Services are going round in circles going nowhere

Over the last 14 years I have attended many meetings, many forums and many stakeholder events and conferences, all of which were used to identify what areas of the mental health services needed to be improved, adapted or developed from the perspective of the people using them and working in them. At the same events, areas for improvement and innovative ideas for the changes needed were made and management thanked us for our input and assured us that these issues would be taken on board and acted upon. Over the last 14 years the same issues have been raised again and again, the same problems highlighted, the same actions needed and the same reassurances given. The actions have not been carried out, the services have not improved and where action has been taken the services have not listened to what people have wanted and they have done what *they* have wanted. Involvement has mainly been tokenistic and where good projects have been carried out the funding has been short-term.

Research projects and evaluations of services are undertaken and again the same issues are highlighted with very few being actioned. Although talking about what needs to be done is a good thing, the services have been doing this as long as I have used them. There needs to come a time when there is *less* talk, *fewer* meetings and *more* action. I have been to some meetings the sole purpose of which has been to arrange other meetings. The core problems are never addressed and the services go round in circles. During the last 14 years the services went from being provided locally to being centralised and now there is talk once again that services need to be provided locally.

Services have been re-amalgamated then spilt up again to provide specific services such as early intervention for psychosis and assertive outreach teams. The core problems are still not addressed. People using the services, in general, always wanted a local service and personally I do not mind if a service is in several small teams or one larger one for my area as long as I get a service that meets my needs. Unfortunately, fragmenting the service as much as they have done means that that there are communication problems between teams and, unless I fit certain criteria or have a specific diagnosis, I do not get the service that best suits me. The limited funding has to be fought for with some services receiving far more than others (especially if they are seen as the 'in thing') and as a result a two-tier service has grown up with some receiving good quality help and support and others not.

Why this is important?

When I needed the support I couldn't get any because the service could not provide what I needed. This meant that I eventually hit crisis point again, which could have been avoided. In the end I asked to be admitted to hospital as I needed the respite and this was the only place that could provide me with any at all, even though hospital was the very last place I wanted to be. I had to practically beg to be admitted but I knew I was in danger of acting on my recurrent suicidal thoughts.

There needs to be action.

Section 3:

Support outside the Mental Health System

Family

Standard Six (*National Mental Health Service Framework, p 69*)
"All individuals who provide regular and substantial care for a person on a CPA should have:

- an assessment of their caring, physical and mental health needs, repeated on at least an annual basis
- their own written care plan which is given to them and implemented in discussion with them"

"In another Social Services Inspectorate report, carers of people with mental health problems were especially critical of how little they were consulted about care plans for service users, how their own needs were not assessed and how little support they received."
(*National Mental Health Service Framwork, p 70*)

Service users and carers themselves indicate that in a crisis they require rapid response, continuity of care and alternatives to hospital-based assessment and admission, such as crisis houses and service user-run sanctuaries in the community.

What do I want from my family?

This is one of the most difficult areas for me. Working with my psychologist has shown me that some of my problems stem from my family relationships. But they are my family and I love them. I want them around me. I need their support. But I also need my independence.

I need their acceptance that I am the way I am, letting me be independent and letting me make my own mistakes, but being there when I need them to be there; having someone to listen unconditionally and being caring and supportive of what I need help with at the time; taking the time to try and understand some of the issues. I don't expect everyone to understand completely but caring enough to want to and supporting my decisions is all I need.

Not being in control of my own life has been made difficult by my family who, although well-meaning and out of love, feel they must over-care and therefore control me. It can make life more difficult when striving for independence. I struggle with saying this because I do need them and love all my family, but sometimes I feel trapped by their love and expectations. I need to make mistakes for myself as I find myself, but I can't do this if wrapped in cotton wool. It must be scary, especially for my parents, to let me go in this way and yes, it's scary for me at times as well. It's safer in that cotton wool.

Happiness is...

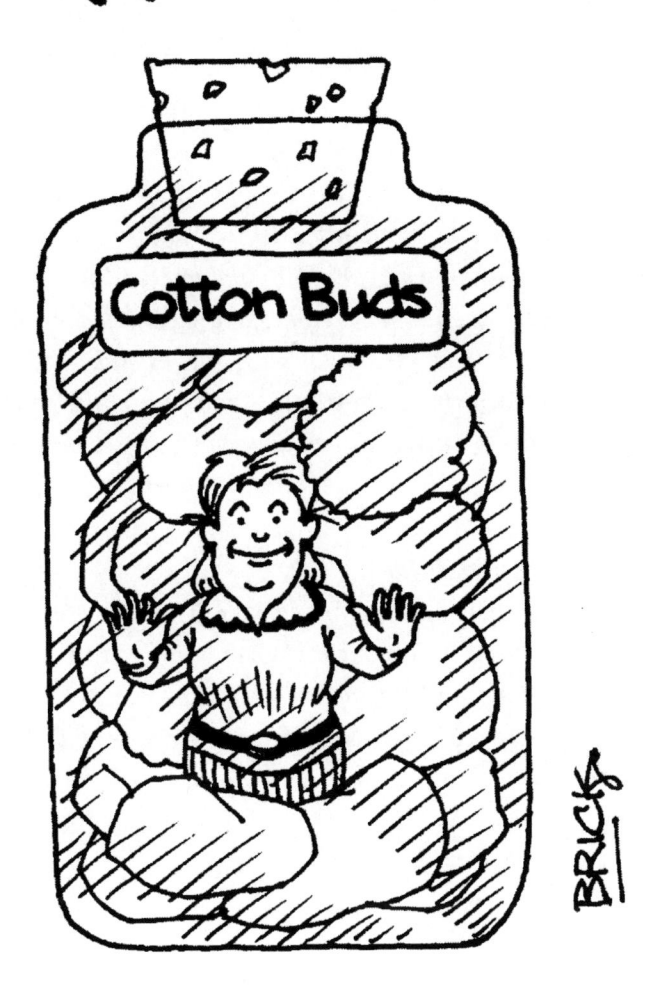

Diary: 23rd November 2003

"I had a dream where I was tied to many bits of rope and elastic of different lengths and thicknesses. At the end of each of the ropes and elastic were different people—my parents, my psychiatrist, my dog, my Gran, other people relating to my mental health, my home, my courses etc. I tried to escape and cut the ties that held me. Some were easy, some were hard and some were so impossible I wasn't strong enough to sever them. I tried then to fly but the few ties that were still attached kept catapulting me back."

Diary: Sunday 7th December 2003

"Some people say I should have a full-time job—a life. Sorry, there is no magic wand. Most days it's hard enough to get up before mid day and on others it's too hard to face the day at all. I can't be like them and having a job for the money isn't that important. I want a life full of love and giving as I receive more in that way. Money does not bring happiness.
I want my parents to be my friends, not my carers".

Diary: 4th February 2004

"I am confused, as when I saw my psychologist again today I talked about my Mum and her need to care for me, Gran and Dad. BUT, then I found I was talking about me and my need to care for others like my Gran. We talked about how my Mum's need for caring was her way of defining herself and in a way it is the same for me. I am more like my Mum than I thought.
The things I've said about her I can say about me and that is scary."

Diary: 10th June 2004

"My psychologist doesn't believe in re-living and examining every detail of your past, but focuses more on what is happening now, though he has used my past experiences to explain the way I am now. It is also the first time my family and the whole dynamic of my social life has been looked at in the entire eight years I have been using the mental health system.

Congruence in today's session was about the way I perceive myself to be. I am an adult with my own belief systems and ideology. I am starting to find out what I want from life, though this is hard. But I am treated by my family as a child and I do admit I feel like a child. And I am treated as not capable not only by my family but also by other professionals involved in my care. It is this mismatch that is partly to blame for my ill health. But how do I escape it?

I feel eleven years old again and I'm re-living the dilemma and torment of then. I was becoming a teenager and I had thoughts and views of my own, but this caused a great deal of tension between me and my Mum. Those endless arguments. My Dad even said to me once, "I know you're right, but for the sake of peace, please apologize to your Mum! For me."

In fact, I apologized so much I became unsure of myself, lost confidence and acquired poor self-esteem. In other ways I tried to rebel, one form of which was the firm stance I took in being a vegetarian. I believed it was right to be vegetarian, but it was also the one thing my family could not stop me from doing and being. It kept me sane, for a while anyway.

The dilemma I face is simple. I could strive and face my fears about going out with the possibility that I will fail or become ill again. That would mean that I would lose any help I have from my parents and on which I'm so reliant at the moment. It would affect the family dynamics and cause distress to my Gran and Dad.

While I am unwell and need support, my Mum is fine. When I become more independent, which includes failing, she doesn't approve. Who would she be if she didn't need to look after us?"

Diary: 02 April 2005

"I had a long session with my psychologist and it overran. I realised in one session the overall dynamics of my situation.

I realised that I was a reflection of Mum. She was angry at others; I am angry at myself. Mum seems not content with others and her life; I am not *content with mine either. She exaggerates every situation; I exaggerate and analyse things inwardly too much.*

I realised I was in the role of a sick person, a patient who needed to be cared for. In my eyes it feels as though both of my parents need me to be in this role for them to feel they are still parents and helping me. It will be hard for them when I break away from the role of sick person and become independent and free.

I realise it's okay for me to be creative and inventive and fun instead of guarding everything I say and do and then analysing everything afterwards. Do other people analyse what they have said?

I shouldn't listen to what my Mum says is right or wrong. I should decide for myself or try it out. If it doesn't work, it doesn't matter."

Both my parents have done the best they can in bringing me up and like all parents they have had their difficulties in doing this. Every generation challenges the last about how their parents parented them. If you had very strict parents you might rebel when you're a parent yourself and be the exact opposite. There will never be a perfect way to bring up a child as so much also depends on the personality of the child itself. All parents will make mistakes and I don't blame my parents for any of them. They did their best for me and I love them for it. I needed the support then and although I viewed it as being wrapped up in cotton wool, overly protected, and was told what I should or shouldn't do, this is what I needed at the time. When I finally started to step out on my own two feet it was very hard for me and my parents to adjust. The roles had become ingrained. Normally a child would become independent before they were twenty; I needed intense support to when I was thirty.

Friends

My friends are still far and few between, but the few I have are real friends and accept me for who I am. I now work as a cubscout leader and have developed a friendship through this that has been my cornerstone for the last two years.

Diary: 15 May 2004

"I spoke to my psychologist about not being able to make friends. I mentioned that when I go to my Chi Yoga all the other people are talking in groups and I am there in a corner not able to think of anything to say, not knowing how to join in. How do you make friends? How do you bond with another human being? Is it something you're born with that I don't have?

He reminded me that I had never formed good relationships as a child, that my best friend was also my bully and that the rest of my friends were much older. I had never had the opportunity to learn the skills as a child that would then come so naturally as an adult.

"How do I begin?" I asked. He said by being more transparent. By being more open to let others in and let them know I struggle. That sometimes I can't pick up the phone, so they will understand when I don't phone them for a while.

Relationships mean commitment and you have to put in to get out. I thought I had been.

Ten minutes later and a bit more harassed I tried to phone a girl I met at a meeting who gave me her number. I waffled on the phone. It was an answer machine and you couldn't re-tape the message. Did I remember to leave my name? I hope she understood me. But I was more transparent because I said I didn't like phones to her in the message."

Grown up in so many ways with an IQ of 124 and still I panic over one simple phone call!

Diary: 2 April 2005

"Today I went on my own with my dog to the local village hall a quarter of a mile away to a coffee morning. I was really anxious and had to stop many times and even spent 10 minutes outside the hall collecting myself.

Luckily for me not many people were there and I got chatting. It was actually nice, although stressful at first as I knew only one person, but then others came. It got busier and in the end about 20 people turned up. I stayed for two cups of tea.

Until I was about twelve I had confidence that I was okay; I need to get back that confidence.

Support groups including peer support

I have received a lot of support from a voluntary organisation (*Framework*) which gave me the practical help I needed to move into a home of my own and become more independent.

I attended a young person's group for a number of years which helped me to develop the basic social skills and support I needed at that time. The safe environment of a group and day centre helped me develop those skills before I was able to move on to do more socially active things in society at large. The group was called *Stepping Stones* and it certainly was a stepping stone for me.

I also started a peer support group because I felt so alone with the experiences I had had on the acute ward and the loneliness of the difficulties I was experiencing at the time. I knew I could not be the only one feeling this way because of the people I had met on the acute ward. I had felt isolated and knew peer support had helped me. I wondered if it could help me in the community as well. I needed people to talk with who had awareness of what I had been through and the distress I was experiencing.

The group has been running 15 years now and I have gained more from it than I have probably given. It has at times kept me out of hospital, kept me from relapsing and supported me from week to week. Knowing you are talking with someone who experiences similar distress is comforting and I can feel safe and secure in talking openly. I have learned from sharing experiences and gained new coping strategies from them.

The group also arranges social activities for its members and this gives us something to look forward to doing together. The support is two-way and this cannot be given by mental health service providers, no matter how much they want to.

The Rushcliffe mental health support group in Nottingham has been essential in my recovery and rediscovery. The group has no professional running it. We are all peers and support each other. We all run the group, some of us more than others, but everyone has a say in how and what we do. Through the group I have learnt to try things out, things like coping strategies that have helped other people. It provides an opportunity to look at the world differently and they always say a problem shared is a problem halved. It is also a social group and I have tried things that I could never do on my own because of my anxieties and fears; but as a group we are stronger. We have met every week, been on outings and even been on holiday. I haven't the strength yet to do this on my own but I am not alone. This is one thing the group has shown me—that I am not alone in my struggles and my fight to survive.

Using our shared knowledge and experience we are able to:
- Collaborate with other organisations to improve the delivery of mental health services and training provision;
- Provide training which informs and empowers mental health service users and carers to have a voice, and enables them to access their rights. This is particularly important when they are sectioned or in hospital;
- Provide a mental health information bank for anybody affected by mental health issues;
- Provide and support opportunities for mental health service

users and carers to get involved, and develop their skills and confidence in meetings and in delivering training.

In 2008 we're hoping to complete a book, written by members of the group, about the value and benefit and the strength our support group gives us.

Activities

Voluntary work and social activities help me by giving me something to look forward to, and purpose and meaning in life. The voluntary work especially does the latter, because it revolves around helping the service to improve and supporting other people who experience distress.

I have recently taken up yoga and although I am not spiritual in that I do not go to church on a regular basis, I have found inner peace. The stretching and gentle exercise has also helped me to feel healthier in myself.

Acupuncture has been very helpful too and has surprisingly beneficial effects. I would never have thought that having needles put into my ears could help me, but it did. It helped by calming my breathing, my thoughts and the hallucinations I was experiencing at the time. I have had a number of auricular acupuncture sessions since this initial session and all have had similar success. These benefits lasted for some considerable time after the session.

Parents' perspective

by David Shaw

There are two words used in this book at which we as Becky's parents take offence—but whoa, we have to be careful! Taking offence at anything will be scrutinised, analysed and have a label put on it, and we will be put in a box, just like Becky. Getting angry would be even worse—we must be guilty of something—one of us might have a personality disorder!

You might gather that we have little time for psychiatrists or the mental health service (apart from a few wonderful exceptions). Like bank managers and doctors, we trusted the service without reservation before we were plunged into its abyss.

What are the offensive words?

"Carers"

Pardon me, we are Becky's parents and all parents are carers—that caring doesn't stop when the child reaches the age of 16 for any parent. Every parent wants the best for their child and has the same worries and aspirations for them whether they are 5 or 35. If a soldier is killed in Iraq they will say on TV news that he was a father of two—not a "carer", no matter how old his sons or daughters are.

"Control"

What an awful word this can seem! Neither of us ever sought to control either of our children, other than to keep them safe.

We believe it is the role of every parent to seek to guide, help, protect, encourage and inspire their children. In our case, these translate as "control". Calling all parents—this applies to you. There is current criticism of parents throughout the country for not giving their children more of a free rein, and millions of children are now tethered to a tight leash by paranoid parents because of the perceived evils of road traffic, muggers, bullies and paedophiles—much more so than we ever tethered our children. If this is the cause of Becky's mental health problems then the services are going to be overwhelmed in a few years' time.

Surely Becky's problems must first and foremost be put down to an unspeakable evil which she seems to have been subjected to when she was very young, a trauma left untreated and unknown, a post-traumatic stress disorder only divulged in Becky's late teens during her first hospital admission, and treated with drugs, not talk. It could be dangerous to talk.

It would also take a lot of professional time and drugs are a lot, lot cheaper!

Our anger and sadness have, to this day, been directed at whoever was responsible for Becky's childhood trauma but we, apparently, should not be doing this. No one knows who was responsible (except perhaps Becky). Nothing will ever be proved and there is no mileage in directing our attentions to that end. We must concentrate on going forward—but we will go back to what we do know and see if the way Becky was spoiled, protected and cared for ("controlled") played a part in the outcome.

We only became aware of a second trauma at the age of 15, when we read this book.

We were no different to any other parents in our village social mix.

Both children went to the local playgroup where Gran helped out. We car-shared the school trips; we enjoyed children's birthday parties with 12–15 local children invited; we spoiled them rotten at Christmas and indeed Becky did stay with Gran for the occasional afternoon or immediately after school until we got back from work.

Yes, we did have concerns about Becky's 'tantrums' but they seemed no more than that—childish tantrums. Yes, we did help and encourage with homework and we did have many family holidays.

Until 12 or 13 Becky was reasonably slim, although big-boned, extremely bright and full of fun. Any parent whose child ballooned to 14 stone at the age of 14 would worry, if not panic. When you see your child is miserable you try to help in any way you can. Is this 'controlling'? Is it wrong?

The dark before the dawn

Becky was admitted to the acute ward at QMC with all the encouragement from her psychiatrist spurring us on,

". . . just a couple of weeks . . . just to get through this crisis"

The dawn before the dark

How little we knew. It had, till then, been comparatively sunny until it went pitch black!

We arrived, Becky terrified, with a case of clothes, and she was admitted to a ward of four patients. We naturally returned the next day to visit and a very smart young lady asked who we wished to see. We explained and she showed us to Becky's room. Even though extremely anxious, Becky was able to tell us that the smart young lady was actually a patient and the nurse was the one with the mini-skirt, halter top and a diamond stud in her navel—it might upset the patients if they wore uniforms—the way you tell is by the ID badge hidden somewhere on them.

After weeks of trying to talk to staff who always said, "in a minute" (they were watching Coronation Street), it started to dawn on us that they had no intention of talking to us. We were not supposed to be there! *We* might be the problem! 'Do they get angry?' 'How are they handling it?' 'Can we give them a label?'
You start to feel more studied than the patient!

Of course, it is most common for a family member to be the abuser—never said, often intimated despite Becky's vehement denials.

What these people could do to us! What power they have!

This appalling unspoken accusation was discussed only once, very calmly. The seething anger inside was kept chained down. "Don't get angry, Dad. It will be misinterpreted. *I* know you never touched me and that's the most important thing."

It's very dangerous to protest or deny to a psychiatrist. In the words of the bard, 'Methinks thou doth protest too much'.

After weeks of asking Becky if staff had talked with her, it also dawned on us that they had no intention of doing that either. They said that Becky had to approach them, which in her state she would not do, so it was just drugs and more drugs (sorry, it's called medication).

Weeks dragged into months while Becky became dopier and dopier. Gradually we were allowed to go on longer walks, then further afield in the car, and eventually she could spend a few nights at home.

When Becky was docile enough (six months later) to be considered no risk to herself, she was discharged into our care. That was the final dawning; it is all about the *elimination of risk* rather than a cure.

The Second Time Around

Becky was admitted to hospital a second time and everything went pretty much as before, right through to the walks in the park and the home visits, until that fateful day when we received a phone call to say Becky had made a suicide attempt on the ward. She had cut her wrists in the toilet and had been there 45 minutes before they found her.

She was put on 'special obs'. This means she was guarded night and day for two weeks, including trips to the toilet or to the shower.

The day after being taken off 'special obs' we were told that she was to be discharged into our care. We were, frankly, terrified. How do we handle the situation? She had been guarded continuously because of the risk and here we were taking on that risk.

We, I think naturally, asked how we were supposed to treat Becky. Should we continuously watch over her? The response was,

"What has it got to do with you?"

Be careful, be calm, don't get angry, that box is beckoning!

As it turned out Becky asked me (Dad) to sleep on the floor next to her bed, which I did every night in a sleeping bag for three months.

When Becky told her psychiatrist of this arrangement his first question was:

"What does he wear when he sleeps next to your bed?"

We understand Becky herself got very angry at that point. Thank you, Becky.

A chink of light

There are more stories, too numerous to tell, which explain our feelings towards the mental health service, but there are people in there who really do care and it was Becky's good fortune to find those who did. Our heartfelt thanks go to those who have taken Becky seriously and seen her potential and have helped her find a strategy for coping and given her a purpose in life. No one can ask more than to have such a purpose.

Determination

Becky was always determined and frankly stubborn in many ways, even as a child.

She could see what was lacking in the Mental Health Care system; namely a forum where people could discuss their problems openly, without fear of deep analysis. She set about forming the Rushcliffe Mental Health Support Group which has gone from strength to strength. It is the mutual support of her own peers which has also gone a very long way in helping Becky feel needed and given her a purpose.

Pride

We have immense pride in what you have achieved, Becky, and you should, too! The best advice you ever had was those 'baby steps'. Just keep taking them and you will get there—or are we 'controlling' you by even just suggesting this?

Conclusion

It may seem as though we have been too harsh in our criticisms of the mental health service. We are certain most doctors and nurses in there are doing what they believe is right for the patient in very difficult and trying circumstances and on very limited budgets. As parents, you rely on any service to do their best for your son or daughter. The service is your only hope and if, in the process, it hurts you, it does not matter as long as it is making your son or daughter well again.

We have never had the opportunity to describe how it feels to us—to give our perspective. Becky's suggestion that we should contribute to this book has provided us with that opportunity. We are grateful for it.

No doubt parents' experiences of the mental health service will not be the same for everyone.

Section 4

Recovery

J.K. Rowling: **"Understanding is the first step to acceptance and only with acceptance can there be recovery."**

Christiaan N. Barnard: **"Suffering isn't ennobling, recovery is."**

"Recovery is about rebuilding a meaningful life, whether or not there are ongoing or recurring symptoms and problems, and whether or not the skills necessary to do everything independently have been acquired. Recovery is not about independence, it is about interdependence, about ensuring that people have access to the supportive relationships they need. Within such a framework, access and inclusion become more important than symptoms and skills."
Repper, J & Perkins, R. (2003).

As I write this book there is a lot of talk about economic recovery. That means the financial world wants the stock market to recover its losses and reach the high peak it's had over the last few years.

The experts tell us that it will be an up-and-down year until we reach that state. That seems an apt simile for recovery if you have mental health problems. Up and down. The graph never stays still, never produces a reassuring straight line across the page.

That's how it is for me. Rather than saying "I've recovered", I'd rather say "I'm in a state of recovery". That state of recovery is an optimistic place for me to be right now. But there is no telling from one day to another the challenges I might have to face, the new things I might have to learn as I explore my current options.

With support I've faced many of the issues of my life and worked through them. I've discovered and learned some coping strategies. I've made that decision to follow my dreams.

But the underlying conditions that I have remain, and will continue to remain. If recovery means the absence of all symptoms, then I agree, I'm not recovered. Just as with malaria you continue to host the conditions to bring on another attack, so I continue to host the conditions to lead to another episode of my problems.

The good news is that I now know it's treatable, manageable and will not stop me living a full life.

It has helped so much seeing a psychologist for two years. He gave me the time and space to work through the emotions of the past before helping me to look at the future. Although he was a psychologist, he was not focused on techniques and fancy methods of intervention or therapy. He was himself and accepted me for myself. He got to know me as an individual and developed a relationship where I could be entirely open and where I felt safe to explore the issues that I needed to work through. I have continued this process through other methods too, like writing, teaching and reflecting.

Diary: October 2004
"After I am gone I wonder who is going to read this and what they will think of me. Will you think of me as a sad and lonely soul with a life that should not have been? I don't want you to feel sorry for me. There have been some great times in this life of mine—a lot of love along with the

heartache. In fact I don't believe you can know what true love is, or have the love without the sadness too. I want you to learn from me, from my experience so that you can help others. I think that is where my compassion comes in, when I do my voluntary work and teaching. I think that is why I am still alive. I don't want you just to listen—I want you to learn and change. I want you to see what my life has been so that you have insight. Then when with others you might be able to think more deeply."

Diary: 22 July 2006

"I haven't written in my diary for a while, well nearly a year. Things have changed a lot. I have someone living with me now. I have made love, which wasn't frightening; it was exhilarating, a release. The tensions and worries in my life are so different from before. I have a life. I am moving forward, and those worries and anxieties that are a part of that life are ordinary. Yes, I still hear voices and at times feel very depressed, but I see the voices more as part of me now, a part of my life. I have my own home—my independence at last. I have purpose again. I start the second part of my degree in January with the Open University and can't wait to complete it.

I am going to do what I always wanted to do, which is become a psychologist. I never thought I could achieve that, and now I know I can. Why not try? What is there to lose? It's the trying that is the fun bit anyway.

If I hadn't tried teaching again I wouldn't have stood up in front of student nurses last week teaching about psychosis. If I hadn't tried living on my own I wouldn't have known I could. If I hadn't tried making love and run away instead, I wouldn't have known how special it could be and would have still been scared to get close to anyone.

Although I dearly want to be with the one I love, I know the time is not ready for him. That time might never come. I know he will always want to stay friends and he will always be a special part of my life. But I am not bound as I was before. I have control over my life at last.

There's something about being bound, then being free, that is an unimaginable experience. Everything is new and exciting to me, like a baby being born to a new world. I caught a train to Edinburgh to see a friend, something I had wanted to do all my life.

Yes, it was frightening to be out in the world on my own but it was great as well: freedom. I can go anywhere now, do nearly anything. What am I going to do? I am going to feel!! Breathe the air, feel the warmth of the sun and say I am glad to be alive.

ME? Who am I? I still don't know, but I do know that I am a warm human being who wants to help others feel the warmth and love that life can bring. I am a lovable, sexual human being who has a lot to give and although I don't know who I am, I have a lifetime to explore that very question.

Am I a jumble of neurons and processors whirring away up there in my brain, or is there more, a soul, a spirit? Is there more to life than carbon and oxygen? I don't know, but I intend to explore and find out. It's the journey, not the answers that I seek.

Every day I am living and learning something new. It feels great to be alive, which is something I thought I never would say. The ups and the downs — well, they are part of that living. Without the downs I wouldn't feel the intense ups, would I?"

Relapse/Crisis

This last year (2007/8) has been hard as both my Grans have died. I have also had to have a huge rethink about my life, partly because of the process of writing this book and the emotional toll that this has taken, and because I finally managed to get to see a psychologist.

During the spring of 2008 I started to go downhill again, I knew I was relapsing as I could see all the signs. I was exhausted but could not rest and because of this my mental health worsened, increasing my hallucinations, depression and the need to keep active all the time to avoid what was going on for me. This could not last, I desperately needed a break otherwise I would crash and be in crisis. My mental health has always been up and down and relapsing at some point was never unavoidable but I knew with the right help I could limit the impact of relapsing and recover more quickly. I needed respite in a supportive environment, to get away from my life, but there was nowhere to go.

In Nottinghamshire there are no respite services only hospital admission for when you are in acute crisis. I needed to avoid hospital as I knew that this would make me worse and my recovery would inevitably take a lot longer. There is no proactive support when relapsing and you can only get support when deep in a crisis. The mental health service is reactive not proactive and this is mainly down to resources and the ingrained negative attitudes of staff and management.

It is well-known by people who regularly use mental health services that if you ask for help in a coherent and logical manner then you won't get the help you need. However if you *show* the services that you need help, especially if you are at risk to yourself, then you will get the help, e.g. rant and rave in public, strip naked and walk the streets, climb on the roof or your house, self harm or attempt suicide (even if you don't want to die but just need help) or something similar.

I have known many, many people who have taken an overdose just to get help even though they may have asked for help just hours before and been fobbed off. Many have also died because of doing this when all they needed was support. I didn't want to do this, even though I have done so in the past, so I asked for help.

I'm trying all the time to balance my need to go forward and learn more, with my need for a stable life and environment. Just as you can have a relapse if you try to do too much physically after a long illness, so it is for me. That means I have to plan carefully what and how much I do.

My main coping strategy when dealing with severe distress, or in relapse, is to take respite. The other thing I do is to talk to someone I trust, before things get out of hand. Currently this is my friend who lives with me, or it can be my community nurse.

When recovering from relapse I take every day as it comes. I congratulate myself for doing something small on days when it is a challenge even to do something small, and challenge myself to something bigger on days when I think I can achieve it. All the time I say to myself, 'I have done it before. I have climbed that mountain and fallen before and climbed again, so I can do it again'.

We all have times when we struggle and we all have different ways of coping. Learning to find those ways of coping and thinking about how to deal with those times is in itself half the battle. When I was first ill I had no coping strategies and little support. Through crisis followed by crisis and through my support group and psychologist, I have learnt different ways that work for me.

At times of severe crisis I have been admitted to hospital. This is not beneficial for me as the acute ward is not a therapeutic place to be and is detrimental to my mental health.

If I had a magic wand I would want somewhere I could go that is peaceful, pleasant, quiet and therapeutic, with people whom I trust, to talk to, and I would receive support not just through medication but from complementary therapies and peer support groups. I would want a tailored approach to my support where I had full say in what would be useful. I would want to be able to access this support *before* I had a crisis not when I was in a crisis, i.e. when I recognised the signs of impending relapse. This would make my recovery time quicker and more successful.

Nigeria—post-traumatic stress—the acute ward

I don't often talk about my experiences in Nigeria, even when asked, as my emotions are still raw. I went out to Nigeria during my third year at university to teach in a summer camp with 8 other people I had never met before arriving at the airport.

After the first few days there was an uprising as the current government imprisoned their newly-elected president. The place I was staying in became a prison. Armed guards on all the gates of the college offered a little more security although this was not much. As I was white and English I was assumed to be rich (even though I was penniless) and we all became a target especially as food and water became scarcer.

Food ran out quickly during that first week and then drinking water also had to be rationed. We would go to the local well and fish out the mud, draining off as much water as we could to use. We had no sterilising equipment but we knew that we had to drink. We all became unwell—most of us had food poisoning, diarrhoea and vomiting. Some had more serious problems which required hospital admission. There were two hospitals, one for paying Nigerians and one for white people (as described by one of the Nigerian teachers). The white hospital was 500 yards down the road and was dangerous to walk to, but this was something we had to do to get the help we needed.

We had few mosquito nets between us and therefore we were bitten alive, with 2 people contracting malaria during the time. We had no proper first-aid kit and even though I had very little first-aid training it was more than anybody else and I therefore became the first-aider. We had no water to wash in or flush the toilets with and in the end we could not use the toilets, opting instead for buckets which we could move our waste away with.

During this time we bonded as a group, working together just to survive. The trip wasn't the best organised in the world in the first place. We had to clean every room when we arrived as we were using a disused college. The college was infested with rats as large as cats. If I had not seen them with my own eyes I would not have believed how big they were or how high those rats could jump. They would pounce onto the mosquito nets as they also were hungry. The cockroaches were commonplace in every room, ranging from lots of tiny ones to huge. I even stood on one for a couple of minutes and when I got off it just wombled away happily. The mattresses were infested with bed mites. The kitchens weren't much better than the rest of the college so we ended up cooking outside on an open fire as it was healthier.

There were many times we had to venture out of the compound to get food and water, try and use a phone or go to the hospital. Many of us, including myself, were held at gun point, saw the bits of bodies beside the road and heard the sounds of gunfire nearby. We all knew people were being killed although at the time it was rarely mentioned between us. There was always a period of unspoken silence after we heard a session of gunfire behind the college.

Sometimes we managed to catch CNN, the only news channel at the hospital, though the reception was poor and intermittent. Deep down we knew how dangerous a situation we were in but we didn't talk about it. Instead we developed a sick sense of humour so as to cope, and concentrated our efforts on survival and eventual escape.

I was lucky in that I had two relatives living and working fairly nearby. I will forever be grateful for their support. They helped us to contact the foreign embassy who could eventually get us out. The British embassy had already gone. The main Nigerian organiser had taken our passports and locked them away and we had to steal them back.

The journey to the airport was nerve-wracking. Five of us managed to get out on the last plane available. There were many other people also trying to get away and only one small plane left. I still feel guilty that I managed to leave. I left behind many Nigerians who had become close friends who I would never see again and I had also left behind the rest of the people with whom I had travelled from the UK (I still don't know if they got back home safely). When I arrived back at Heathrow I resisted the urge to kiss the ground beneath me and clung to my Dad. It was from then that I crumbled and the reality of what I had been through struck me.

When I got home my parents said I could have anything I wanted to eat—takeaway pizza, Chinese—anything. All I wanted was baked beans on toast and a fresh glass of water. It was the best meal I have ever had, even though I still couldn't eat much.

Although very different in many respects, I liken the after-effects of my time in Lagos in Nigeria to my experience of being on the acute ward. The bonding with others in my group that I experienced in Nigeria was similar to that of the bonding I had with other patients on the ward. We had to support each other. We developed the same sense of humour in order to cope.

The sub-culture that developed in both Nigeria and on the ward was again similar. Being on an acute ward has its own unique culture and is very different to ordinary society. It has its own unwritten rules, ways of working and hierarchical structure. The main similarity was the lack of power and control in both situations. In Nigeria it was slightly easier as we could fight for some control over what happened to us, but on a ward you can't. The wards are locked and the decisions made about you are remote from you.

The main similarity, though, was that I came away from Nigeria and the acute ward with the same symptoms of post-traumatic stress.

When I left the ward after six months of being an inpatient, coming out into the real world was a shock. Noises were overwhelming, especially traffic, colours were brighter, air was cooler and breathtaking and the world seemed busier. Every one of my senses was over-stimulated. I wanted to go back in! It was horrible and scary but at the same time it was wonderful as it meant freedom. After both my time in Nigeria and on the acute ward I then had to relearn how to live. I was anxious about everything that I did—cooking, cleaning and other daily tasks, but especially going out and being with people. I had difficulty making decisions for myself. In some respects Nigeria was easier to cope with as I was now completely away from the situation. But coming from the acute ward back into the community meant the mental health services still controlled me, decisions were made for me and there was always the threat that I could be put back there again if I didn't comply.

I did learn one crucial thing from my experiences in Nigeria that has helped me in my recovery from mental health difficulties and that is, if you had told me before I went that I would go through that experience I would not have believed that I could cope so well. I discovered I had strength inside me that I never thought possible. I had the ability to adapt and cope with what I previously would have thought was impossible. I can do what I believed I couldn't.

Accepting failure and rejection as part of recovery

I understand who I am and accept the difficulties I face, but I know now that it should not stop me from being open with others about my mental health, even with the fear I have of possible rejection.

People get rejected all the time, for many reasons, and it can be hard sometimes to face the fact that not everyone is going to like you as a person. But I have accepted that. It is great that we are all unique individuals and a diverse species. It's what makes us human and gives us strength and because I no longer fear being open, I have found I am no longer as paranoid about people finding out about my mental health difficulties as I was when I tried to hide them.

I have found that it wasn't as bad as I expected, and that being open has in fact intrigued people and helped them to also open up about themselves. I still get some people who don't want to know and some who are prejudiced, but letting people get to know me, and being open, has gone some way to dismissing the myths surrounding mental health.

Accepting myself for who I am also helped me when I became visually impaired five years ago. I used the very same philosophy of adaptation and acceptance and the belief that I could continue to live a full and meaningful life, just as I have done with my mental health difficulties.

At the moment I am happy with who I am, but it has not always been that way, as this book shows. By telling my story here I am hoping that others can realise there is always light at the end of the tunnel, however far away it might seem at times. It is also my fervent hope that my experiences recounted here will be useful to them.

What can you do to help?

Whether you are a mental health worker, psychiatrist, psychologist or Joe Bloggs down the road, just treat me how you yourself would want to be treated. You have made a start by reading this book.

It doesn't take fancy degrees to help me. In fact, quite the opposite. It takes someone who cares, really cares, and cares not for the money but who would behave the same whether they were being paid or not. In any case, very few people go into the mental health services for the money—or the glory!

It requires a frame of mind like the cleaner who worked on the acute ward during my first admission, who was straightforward and just herself. Having people around me who are honest, caring, want to help, even with the practical things (which can seem to be the biggest hurdles of all) can be, and are, of far greater value to me than some of the trained professionals.

You may feel a horror of 'those people' but take a moment to think how you'd react if you had to watch someone you love descend into a depressive state, or start to do strange things.

Some of the behaviours exhibited by people experiencing mental health distress, viewed from the outside can seem strange. To the person, their actions at the time have their own internal logic; it just isn't obvious to the outsider.

Even people who don't react badly to mental health sufferers can behave in an odd way. For instance, I was talking to a man where I help out as a volunteer. When he realised I had mental health difficulties, he started to speak slowly and didn't even know he was doing it!

How I see my future now

Although I don't know what my future holds for certain, I do know that I will continue on this journey of discovery for the whole of my life.

As well as a small amount of teaching, I am now undertaking a part-time, distance-learning degree. This is something I have wanted to do for a long time and which I can do, with support, when at home and unable to go out. Studying for the degree means I am developing new skills and challenging myself, and it is also something I am in control of, as I often need to take time out and can only work in very small bursts.

Most of all I have grown as a person to a new level of awareness. Deep depression is awful and I cannot describe how lonely that pit of despair is every time I go through it, but coming out of that depression is like being awake for the first time. Everything is colourful again and sounds are brighter. I live for that time. The hallucinations too have their good points, even in the darkest times, as some of these experiences are insightful and even, on occasion, beautiful.

I would not like anyone to go through what I have been through during the last 30 years, but it has had some benefits. I have gained a unique awareness about myself and the experiences of other people who have gone through similar rough times. I am more empathetic and aware of my emotions. I have changed the direction my life was taking and, although I have come full circle back to teaching, I have had a life experience that no one can take from me, which informs and empowers me at the same time.

Making new friends who accept me for who I am is invaluable and I do believe I would not have gained these friendships without the experiences I have had. I now have a new drive and motivation to work with the mental health services with the aim of improving them.

You might ask, what has this to do with my recovery? Well, lots!! Take the situation many of us with mental problems are in, of being on benefits. Personally, I hate it. I would much rather work, but I can't. I need to access benefits to live. The pressure that society puts on people like me to force us to work has made me ill more than once. There was a time when I deliberately came off benefits, built myself up to undertake employment and made an attempt at paid work. I quickly ended up back in hospital. Most of us use the system because we need to, not because we want to be a drain on society or abuse the system in any way. These suspicions and pressures make us feel devalued and deflated, leaving us with low morale, low self-esteem and an increased likelihood of relapse.

The benefits system treats us as criminals, guilty until proven innocent. I understand that they have to make sure people aren't cheating, but the forms are extremely complicated and when you are feeling ill at the time it's very easy to make mistakes.

For my voluntary work I teach students and mental health staff by giving them the benefits of my real-life experiences in using the mental health system, and inspiring them to *see past the label and recognise the individual*. I am hopeful this will eventually lead to real service improvements. I am highly motivated to this end because I have had some particularly bad experiences using the services and I want to do something about this to help make a better future for all mental health sufferers.

I have spent a lifetime hiding my feelings both from myself and other people and this has only made me feel worse. I have spent my whole life trying to be what other people wanted me to be—or what I thought they wanted me to be.

It doesn't matter what people think about me anymore. Yes, I would like everyone to like me and yes, occasionally it hurts, being excluded because of my label, but I just tell myself that I can't help what people think of me. I am me and nothing is going to change that and I wouldn't want to be anyone else. I may have my problems. I may still do and say the wrong things at times, but this is something we all do at some point in our lives. I am still happy with me. How many of us can say that? I can't change how other people think or act, but I can take responsibility for what *I* think and do.

It has helped others when they have heard the story of my journey and I hope that, now you have read it too, it will have given *you* a better understanding of just one life lived with mental health problems. I hope that you now have a clearer picture of the difficulties faced by mental health sufferers, and I also hope it has inspired you that people can live full lives, even within the shadow of the difficulties they face.

Recovery is possible

There is no one definition of recovery, there never can be. It is the individual who defines it, the individual who owns it. The journey out of the tunnel belongs to the individual alone.

I live with my voices and the ups and downs as a part of my life. Living with these experiences and managing them in the best way I can is important. I may never be free of them but *I can still live a full and meaningful life*. This gradual but oh so important realisation has been the recovery or rediscovery I needed. I now live for me and every day I say to myself that if I want to do something, then why not? It might take me longer or I might need to do it in a different way, but I can still do it. Just like the person in a wheelchair who adapts and isn't ruled by the boundaries their disability could impose, so am I not bound by the supposed limitations of my mental health.

I used to feel imprisoned by the effects of experiencing frequent and recurrent distress and the unusual experiences that were part of my every day. Added to this, the treatment I received for a long time told me over and over that I was ill and would be ill for life and that I could not recover. Realising that *this isn't true*, that my life can in fact be meaningful and fulfilling, that I may not always be a mental health service user, and finding myself and following my dreams, I have stepped off that treadmill and now have a life to live.

I am Becky, and society can either accept me, or not, but I am not going to change simply because society cannot tolerate difference: nor should you. Recovery has been about finding myself and rediscovering not what is important to others but what is important to *me*.

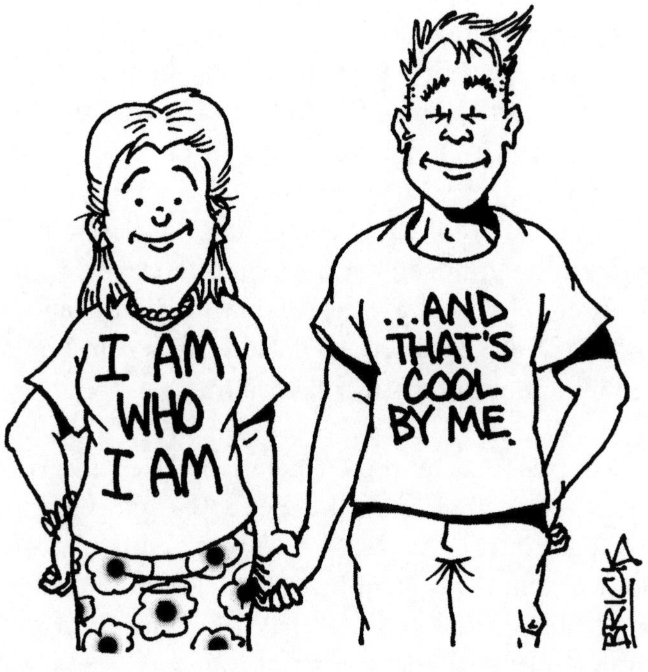
I AM WHO I AM
...AND THAT'S COOL BY ME.
BRICK

Final tips

1. You only get one life. Live it. Discover what you want to get out of it and say to yourself, Why not! Then do it for you.

2. Life has it ups and downs, its thrills and spills, but it's just a ride. Enjoy it, and remember that you can get through the downs no matter how dark they seem at the time. And don't forget—praise yourself *each step* of the way!

3. Don't blame yourself either. We can all look back with hindsight. We all make mistakes. We are all human. But we can learn from them and move forward. I spent my life looking at what I couldn't do instead of looking at what I could. The moment I started to realise I *could* do things was the moment I discovered *more* of what I could do.

4. Take control as you only get one chance at life. Get support in doing this as you will find great value in having like minds together.

5. Talk to and be with your peers. Having people around you who understand and empathise, who are honest and trustworthy, is essential for your well-being.

Visions

In this book I've talked about my experiences in the mental health service and I've also talked about how I, as a service user, think it can be improved.

In order to improve anything we need a vision of how it should be. I'd like to finish by using this quotation from someone who is both a service user and a worker. I share her vision.

"I have a vision:

That those of us with mental health problems can be known for the contribution we make to our communities—celebrated for our heroes rather than derided or feared because of our villains:

That we can end the national disgrace that 87% of people who experience mental health problems are unemployed:

That one day I will be able to talk about my mental health problems and attract no more than interest in those around me; that one day we will see a prime minister who openly talks about his or her experience of mental health problems:

That mental health services will focus more on our abilities than our disabilities, helping us grow, develop, pursue our lives:

That having people with mental health problems providing mental health services will be no more unusual than the numerous professionals working in general hospitals and primary care who have physical illnesses:

Finally, I have a vision that those of us with mental health problems will be able to talk of our visions without them being written of as 'delusions', 'lack of insight', 'unrealistic'. I have a vision that my visions will be taken seriously."

Dr Rachel Perkins – service user, clinical psychologist and mental health manager, *Openmind*, 104, July/August 2000, page 6.

Section 5

Glossary

In this glossary section I've put some more definitions (including abbreviations). Professionals often talk in abbreviations, assuming you understand.

Advocate
A person who speaks on behalf of another.

Carer
A person who supports someone else. Could be a family member or friend.

Citizens Advice
Citizens Advice Bureaux are available in most areas. They offer impartial advice. For information on your own area see their entry in your local phone book.

Cognitive Behaviour Therapy(CBT)
What is CBT? CBT can help you to change how you think ("Cognitive") and what you do ("Behaviour)". These changes can help you to feel better. Unlike some of the other talking treatments, it focuses on the "here and now" problems and difficulties. Instead of focusing on the causes of your distress or symptoms in the past, it looks for ways to improve your state of mind now.

Community mental health nurses (CMHN)
CHMNs are also known as CPNs (Community Psychiatric Nurses). They work as part of a community mental health team often based at GP surgeries. They can have specialist areas of experience such as children, elderly people, drug or alcohol problems.

Community Mental Health Team (CMHT)
CMHTs are found in each local area where they support people with longer-term mental health difficulties within the community. Support is offered by psychiatrists, nurses, occupational therapists, social workers and other mental health workers.

Counsellor
Counselling is described as a 'talking' treatment. It can help people manage a wide range of problems. Access to counselling services can be difficult to arrange in the NHS.

Gateway worker
A recent addition to mental health services providing a similar form of assessment as admission nurses in accident and emergency units.

General practitioner (GP)
Can be the first point of contact for many patients. They can work singly or as part of a multi-agency team providing mental health care.

Health visitor
Can offer advice on general health with special training in child health.

Healthcare Commission
This body assesses the effectiveness of services delivered by the NHS. As part of its role it carries out surveys of mental health services including surveying patient feedback.

Occupational Therapists
They work within the community, day hospitals and secure psychiatric units. Their work is based on helping individuals become more confident and build skills needed to live in the community. They also focus on anxiety management and assertiveness training.

Patient Advice and Liaison Services (PALS)
Part of their functions was previously run by community health councils. PALS are established in each NHS Trust and work to help patients sort out treatment problems within that Trust. Any problem they can't solve within the Trust will probably be referred to:

Independent Complaints Advocacy Service (ICAS)
ICAS is a service independent to the NHS which helps service users or their carers to pursue a complaint about treatment.

Patient and Public Involvement (PPI) forums
PPI forums are available in each NHS Trust. However they don't become involved in individual treatment issues but work to improve services based on feedback from the community.

Peer support groups
A peer is someone who is an equal, with similar social power and knowledge. A peer support group is composed of individuals who see each other as equals. Peer support works because it is a two-way process. Decisions can be made by the entire group. Being a member of a peer support group can validate and give confidence to individuals who feel disempowered in other situations.

Psychiatrist
Psychiatrists are medically trained doctors who have specialised in mental health. They can work in hospitals, the community as part of multi-agency teams, or individual secure units.

Psychologists
Unlike psychiatrists, psychologists do not have to be medically trained. They must have a degree in psychology plus work experience. They can further qualify by studying a particular type of psychology such as clinical psychology or counselling psychology.

Psychotherapist
A psychotherapist may be a psychiatrist, a psychologist or other mental health professional with special training.
Psychotherapy works to find our why you feel as you do and why you respond to others the way you do.

Social workers
Social workers offer support for a variety of social rather than medical needs, and not only within mental health.

Approved Social Worker
Approved social workers (ASW) have been trained in specific functions under the Mental Health Act (1983).

Section 6

Resources

There are many websites and books available on mental health issues. I encourage you to read widely but please read with caution. There is much information which is misleading, unhelpful and wrong. The resources in this section have been chosen with care to reflect policy, needs and experiences.

If you need help, look for a local peer-support group as its members have first hand experience of the problems you face. If you are considering withdrawing from medication always get support. It isn't something to do lightly.

The list I've included is not exhaustive—we could have filled a book with information about resources. I've included some I've used in the Nottingham area and some national ones. In your area you may find them advertised in your surgery, library, mental health team bases and local voluntary services.

Books

Veronica Decides to Die' by Paul Coehlo is a book I would recommend anyone to read who wants to know from the inside what it feels like to think about suicide.

Ron Coleman *'Working to Recovery'* are books and training for voice-hearers, trainers and service users. www.workingtorecovery.co.uk

Organisations

Contact information about the following organizations has been taken from their websites. The information was correct at the time of going to press.

Citizens Advice Bureau
This is a general help and advice service. For contact details in your area please check in your local phone book or Yellow Pages.

Depression Alliance
http://www.depressionalliance.org/docs/what_we_offer/self_help_groups.html
For an information pack you can telephone 0845 123 23 20 or send an email to information@depressionalliance.org or write to:
Depression Alliance
212 Spitfire Studios
63 - 71 Collier Street
London N1 9BE

Eating Disorders Association
beat is the **beat** is the working name of the Eating Disorders Association and is the leading UK charity for people with eating disorders and their families.
103 Prince of Wales Road, Norwich, NR1 1DW
Helpline: 0845 634 1414   E-mail: help@b-eat.co.uk
beat Youthline: 0845 634 7650   E-mail: fyp@b-eat.co.uk
www.b-eat.co.uk

Hearing Voices Network
79 Lever Street. Manchester M1 1FL
Enquiries and information: 0845 122 8641
Email: info@hearing-voices.org   Website: www.hearing-voices.org

Kidscape
Kidscape is committed to keeping children safe from abuse.
Kidscape, 2 Grosvenor Gardens, London SW1W 0DH.
Telephone: 020 7730 3300 Fax: 020 7730 7081
Helpline: 08451 205 204
The helpline is for the use of parents, guardians or concerned relatives and friends of bullied children. If you are a child and are experiencing bullying problems, ring **Childline** 0800 1111

MHHE
www.headacademy.ac.uk
Enhancing learning and teaching about mental health in Higher Education.

The Mental Health Foundation
Founded in 1949, the Mental Health Foundation is a leading UK charity that provides information, carries out research, campaigns and works to improve services for anyone affected by mental health problems, whatever their age and wherever they live.
Mental Health Foundation, London Office, 9th Floor, Sea Containers House, 20 Upper Ground, London, SE1 9QB
Telephone: 020 7803 1101 Fax 020 7803 1111
Email: mhf@mhf.org.uk
www.mentalhealth.org.uk

MIND
MIND is a national charity providing a variety of services. These include day centres and phone support lines to help those who have mental health problems and also their supporters, families and carers.
For all their services go to www.mind.org.uk
Telephone helpline 0845 766 0163

NAPAC(National Association for People Abused in Childhood)
All correspondence NAPAC receives is treated with the strictest confidentiality, but if given information which is considered to disclose current incidences of abuse, the appropriate authorities will be informed.
Telephone: 0208 974 68 14 (open 10am to 3pm Monday, Wednesday & Friday; 10am to 1pm Tuesday & Thursday)
E-mail: advice@rethink.org
If you are an adult survivor of child abuse and require support, information or advice, please contact at: 42 Curtain Road, London EC2A 3NH
Support Line 0800 085 3330

National Self-Harm Network
The National Self-Harm Network (UK based but available to everyone from ANY country) has been a survivor-led organisation since 1994. It consists of committed campaigners for the rights and understanding of people who self-harm.
NSHN, PO Box 7264, Nottingham NG1 6WJ

National Service User Network
The National Survivor User Network (NSUN) brings together groups and organisations in England, that are run by users and survivors of mental health services, into one national network.
27-29 Vauxhall Grove, Vauxhall, London SW8 1SY
Telephone: 0845 602 0779
Email: info@nsun.org.uk   www.sustn.net

NHS Direct
www.nhsdirect.nhs.uk
In the search box on the left-hand side of the site, type in mental health services. The page which comes up has links to support services on the right-hand side of the page.

Rethink
"Working together to help everyone affected by severe mental illness recover a better quality of life."
www.rethink.org   Email: info@rethink.org
Rethink Head Office, 5th Floor, Royal London House, 22-25 Finsbury Square, London EC2A 1DX
Telephone: 0845 456 0455

Sainsbury Centre for Mental Health
134-138 Borough High Street, London SE1 1LB
Tel: 020 7827 8300   Fax: 020 7827 8369
Email: contact@scmh.org.uk
They provide information and carry out research

Samaritans
www.samaritans.org.uk
Samaritans provide a 24 hour support line.
Tel: 0847 767 8000

SANELINE
SANELINE provides a telephone helpline giving practical information, emotional support and crisis care for those with mental health problems.
SANE, 1st Floor Cityside House, 40 Adler Street London E1 1EE
E-mail: info@sane.org.uk
Telephone: 020 7375 1002   Fax: 020 7375 2162
Website: www.sane.org.uk
SANEline: 0845 767 8000
SANEmail: sanemail@sane.org.uk

SUSTN Service User Survivor Trainer Network
SUSTN is a new national network that aims to support service users who are now providing mental health training
www.sustn.net

UK Mental Health Research Network

The UK Mental Health Research Network (MHRN) is funded by the Department of Health and was established to provide the NHS infrastructure to support both non-commercial and commercial large-scale research in mental health, including clinical trials. It is one of the topic-specific networks under the umbrella of the UK Clinical Research Network (UKCRN) and is managed by a partnership between the Institute of Psychiatry, King's College, London and the University of Manchester.

PO Box 77, Institute of Psychiatry, Kings College London, De Crespigny Park, London SE5 8AF
Telephone: 020 7848 0699   Fax: 020 7848 0696
Email: mhrn@iop.kcl.ac.uk

East Midlands Hub, MHRN
Email: ann.priddey@nottingham.ac.uk
B21 Gateway Building
University of Nottingham Innovation Park
Triumph Road, Nottingham
NG7 2TU

Witness

Witness is dedicated to helping people who have been abused by health and social care workers and works to prevent abuse. This is done by providing a helpline and professional support and advocacy services for the victims and survivors of abuse, and by campaigning for improvements in policy law and practice, conducting research and providing education and training.
32-36 Loman Street, London SE1 0EE
Helpline 08454 500 300
Email: info@witnessagainstabuse.org.uk

Rebecca Shaw publications

Roberts S, Collier R, Shaw B, Cook J, (2007) *Making Waves in Nurse Education: The PINE Project in* Stickley T, Basset T (eds.) *Teaching Mental Health.* 9-27, Chichester: Wiley

Houghton P, Shaw B, Hayward M, West S, (2006) Psychosis Revisited: Taking a collaborative look at psychosis, *Mental Health Practice 9,* pp 40-43

Shaw R, (2007) 'Cutting the path', *INVOLVE Newsletter,* Autumn: 1-3

Stickley T, Shaw R, (2006) Evaluating social inclusion, *Mental Health Practice, Volume 9 No 10 July*

References

Basset, T., Cooke, A., & Reid, J. (2003) *Psychosis Revisited: a workshop for mental health workers*; order from Pavilion Publishing Tel: 01273 623222, www.pavpub.com,

Bazelon Center for Mental Health Law (2004) *Get it together: how to integrate physical and mental health care for people with serious mental disorders*; www.bazelon.org

British Psychological Society. (2000). *Recent advances in understanding mental illness and psychotic experiences. A report by the British Psychological Society Division of Clinical Psychology;* The British Psychological Society
Note. This document can be downloaded at www.understandingpsychosis.com

Elliott, Jane (1960s) *Blue eyes experiment* an elementary school teacher; Iowa

Elliott, Jane – see www.janeelliott.com for more information

Hatloy, I MIND (2008) *Statistics 1 Fact sheet*; MIND Broadway London, UK www.mind.org.uk

Northfield, J (2004) *Factsheet – what is a learning disability? B.I.L.D*; British Institute of Learning Disabilities, Kidderminster

Rosenhan, D.L (1973) *On being sane in insane place;* Science, 179, 250-58

Repper, J & Perkins, R. (2003). *Social inclusion and Recovery: A Model for Mental Health Practice;* Balliere Tindall.

Perkins, Rachel, (2000) *Openmind*; Issue 104, page 6, (for more information see www.mind.org)

Slade, P.D. and Bentall, R.P. (1988) *Towards a scientific analysis of hallucination*; London, Croom Helm.

Stewart, G MIND (2007) *Understanding mental illness booklet*; MIND Broadway London, UK www.mind.org.uk

Tien, A.Y.(1991) *Distributions of hallucinations in the population*; Social Psychiatry and Psychiatric Epidemiology, 26, 287-292.

Other References

(20 March 2000) No Secrets; Department of Health and Home Office

(1983, last modified 9 February 2007) *1983 Mental Health Act*; The Stationery Office

World Health Report 1999; as quoted from National Mental Health service Framework

(September 1999) *National Mental Health Service Framework;* Department of Health

Rollo May Love and Will (2007) *depression reference*; W W Norton

Why I need to publish this book

I am fearful of publishing this book and I need to express why.

Mental health difficulties are hidden and the fear surrounding people who have these difficulties is greater because their experiences are largely unfamiliar to and not talked about by the general public.

There are a lot of people who already know me and not only because of my role within mental health services or from my work with the support group. Some of these people will not even know that I *have* a mental health history or current difficulties, and they may not know much about mental health either.

I am exposing my inner self to you in what I have written.

I hope that you will respond positively and will be able to see the benefits of writing this book. Some elements of my life came as a shock even to my own parents when they read the draft of the book, but it has helped us to talk more openly about the difficulties I have faced and the challenges that my parents have also had to deal with.

One in four people will experience mental health problems every year and you may know people close to you—friends, family, colleagues—who struggle. The only way to tackle the stigma that surrounds mental health is by talking about it, freely and easily. Many of my friends feel they cannot talk about their difficulties with anyone at all, which leaves them feeling isolated and anxious and frightened that if they do they will be treated differently and not as part of mainstream society. I have to acknowledge that this is a real and constant fear. Opening myself to you and publishing this book is my way of challenging the prejudice that is out there.

It is my burning hope that through reading this book other people will feel able to be more open about the mental health difficulties they face.

I know already the effect that reading this book has had on my parents. They have learnt new things about me and it has meant we have talked more openly about my treatment and about their experiences of the service. I want to give comfort to those going through similar difficulties by showing them that they, like me, can get through and live a meaningful life. For people who have not experienced mental health distress I want to increase awareness about what it is like for the individual sufferer, what helps and what hinders.

This book will inevitably stimulate conversation and debate about mental health and the way people are supported. It will tell you what the mental health services are really all about and what in an ideal future they could become.

This book is going to be widely available and if you already know me, when you have read it you may perceive me in a very different way. What will you think of me? Will what I have written be understood or misinterpreted? Will you react to me differently? Will you avoid me? Will you discriminate against me?

I don't know the answers to any of the above. I do know that I am going to publish this book and I will face and deal with the answers as they come along.

I hope you understand.

Becky

DISCOVERING RECOVERY
From Mental Health Distress

The experiences of a mental health
support group

About this book:

We are writing this book so that we can share our learning from several areas.

- Firstly, to share the effect that the experience of a small support group can have on individuals
- Secondly, to share our experiences of what helps and what doesn't help when experiencing mental health distress
- Thirdly, to tell you about group members' individual experiences of mental health services

Finally, the aim of the entire book is to highlight *the recovery process* from mental health distress. It offers hope and optimism for those currently in distress, and tips for those people supporting them.

"The journey to recovery is an ongoing path of discovery. All the contributors to this book are at different stages of their journey."

Becky Shaw (founder)
bshawmh@inbox.com